Diagnosis and Management of Poisoning

JK Grover
Ex-Professor and Head
Department of Pharmacology
All India Institute of Medical Sciences
New Delhi

Monica Malik

PEEPEE
PUBLISHERS AND DISTRIBUTORS (P) LTD.

Diagnosis and Management of Poisoning

Published by
Pawaninder P. Vij

Peepee Publishers and Distributors (P) Ltd.
Head Office: 160, Shakti Vihar, Pitam Pura
Delhi-110 034 (India)

Corporate Office: 7/31, Ansari Road, Daryaganj
Post Box-7243, New Delhi-110002 (India)

Ph: 55195868, 23246245, 9811156083

e-mail: peepee160@yahoo.co.in

e-mail: peepee160@rediffmail.com

e-mail: peepee160@gmail.com

www.peepeepub.com

First Edition: **2006**

ISBN: 81-88867-90-X

Printed at:
Lordson, C-5/19, Rana Pratap Bagh, Delhi-110 007

Preface

Today there is a wide variety of toxic substances—both natural and man made—that are harmful to humans worldwide, over the years, there has been an increase in mortality and morbidity due to toxins. However, this fact is yet to be appreciated in India. A large proportion of the Indian population lives in villages which have their own unique problems as regards toxic substances. Signs and symptoms of poisoning may often be confused with many other clinical conditions unless there is high index of suspicion. Unfortunately accurate diagnosis and treatment is often delayed or completely lacking due to lack of awareness and infrastructures.

With this book, we aim to fill these voids that exist in our country today as regards diagnosis and management of poisoning. Although there are a few books on the subject, none are specific to the Indian context. A unique feature of this book is that it has comprehensively covered a wide spectrum of poisonous substances including chemicals, drugs, household items and toxins of plant and animal origin. We have included the associated clinical signs and symptoms and the laboratory investigations which assist in arriving at proper diagnosis. In addition we have tried to comprehensively address various issues in management including specific antidotes along with their doses and route of administration, monitoring of patients during therapy and supportive care. Therefore, this book will be useful for medical practitioners, students and paramedical staff and has been designed in a simple and easy to understand format keeping in mind the specific needs of all these groups.

JK Grover
M Malik

Contents

G

GAMMAXINE

It is usually used as insecticide in agriculture and as 1% solution for the treatment of scabies and pediculosis.

Symptoms

Unconsciousness and myoclonus.

Muscle tone is greatly increased and reflexes are exaggerated.

Vomiting, convulsions, rhabdomylosis, severe acidosis and disseminated intravascular coagulation are other features associated with gammaxine toxicity.

Renal tubular and hepatocellular necrosis, pancreatitis and proximal myopathy with myoglobinuria have been reported.

Polymorph leukocytosis, increased serum aspartate aminotransferase and lactic dehydrogenase may be present.

Management

No specific treatment.

General measures include emptying of stomach (if the case is presented within 4 hours of ingestion of the poison), arterial blood gas analysis followed by correction of acid base abnormality.

Convulsions require treatment by curarization and mechanical ventilation only if frequent.

Supportive and symptomatic treatment needs to be followed.

GANJAH

It is flowering stalk of female plants. It is usually smoked in pipe (chilm) and is less potent than charas but more potent than bhang. Fatal dose is 8 gm/kg body weight.

Clinical Picture

Same as with other **Cannabis indica** *(Refer page 90)*.

Treatment

Same as with other **Cannabis** *(Refer page 90)*.

GASES IRRITANT (Ammonia, Hydrogen Chloride Phosgene)

G

A vast number of compounds produce irritant effects when inhaled in their gaseous form. The most common source of exposure to irritant gases is in industry but significant exposure may occur in a variety of circumstances such as after mixing cleaning agents at home.

Symptoms

Low level exposure causes irritation of mucous membranes and upper respiratory tract, conjunctivitis, rhinitis, skin erythema and burns. Sore throat, cough, wheezing and hoarseness are common. Symptoms are rapid in onset.

With high level exposure, laryngeal edema, tracheobronchitis and abrupt airway obstruction may occur. Irritation of the lower respiratory tract and lung parenchyma may cause tracheobronchial mucosal sloughing, chemical pneumonitis and non-cardiogenic pulmonary edema.

Management

Remove victim from area of contamination and give supplemental oxygen if needed. Rescuers should take care to avoid personal exposure.

There is **no specific antidote** for any of these gases and therefore poisoning is treated symptomatically.

Hoarseness or stridor suggests laryngeal edema that requires laryngoscopy and endotracheal intubation. Assist ventilation if necessary.

Give supplemental oxygen and treat bronchospasm with aerosolized bronchodilators.

Monitor arterial blood gases, chest X-ray and pulmonary functions. Treat pulmonary edema if present.

For victims of smoke inhalation, consider the possibility of concurrent intoxication by carbon monoxide or cyanide.

GASOLINE (Petrol)

Gasoline (petrol): Naphta, mineral spirits, kerosene and other aliphatic hydrocarbons are petroleum distillates and are poorly absorbed from the GIT.

Gasoline and naphtha are highly volatile and inhalation of fumes can cause CNS depression even if pulmonary toxicity is not manifested.

There is high risk of aspiration pneumonia.

Toxic dose: It is difficult to determine the exact dose but in experimental animals 1 ml when introduced into the pulmonary tract can cause toxicity.

Symptoms of Toxicity

Vomiting is common but not necessary. Diarrhoea is uncommon.

There may be excitement, but in severe poisoning drowsiness is seen which may lead to coma.

The most common complication of this poisoning is pulmonary troubles which occur in almost 60% resulting into cough, choking, wheezing and breathlessness.

Clinically respiratory involvement is usually evident within few moments after exposure but in some cases it may be delayed for hours (but never more than a day). Severe poisoning can cause hemorrhagic pulmonary oedema which is fatal within 24 hours. Pneumonitis in most of the cases involves two or more lobes and is peripheral in distribution. Fever and polymorph leukocytosis are common.

Rare complications include development of pneumatocele, intravascular hemolysis and renal failure.

Management

Gastric emptying is favoured specially if sufficiently large amount of the poison has been ingested. However this can be undertaken only if the patient is sufficiently alert so that he can cough effectively and second the airway should be protected by cuffed endotracheal intubation.

If signs of serious poisoning are evident, gastric emptying is indicated.

Antibiotics should be given in only those patients who develop secondary bacterial infections.

If cyanosis is present, oxygen may be necessary. Intermittant positive pressure is indicated for patients with pulmonary oedema.

GELSEMIUM (Yellow Jessamine)

It is woody climbing vine with paired, lance-like leaves and clusters of funnel shaped yellow flowers.

All parts of the plant are toxic:

The roots being most toxic.

Toxicity is due to presence of three alkaloids-gelsemoidin. These alkaloids interfere with cholinergic transmission at neuromuscular junction and CNS by binding to acetylcholine receptors.

Symptoms of Toxicity

G

Headache, vertigo, blurred vision, mydriases, nausea, dysphagia, muscular weakness and collapse.

Management

Stomach wash followed by activated charcoal.

Remaining management same as for **Atropine** *(Refer page 68).*

GINSENG (Plant)

Root of this deciduous perennial plant (Panax ginseng) is used medicinally in treatment of CNS disorders, fatigue and impotence. Panaxin, panax acid, paraquilin and ginsenin are the active principles.

Symptoms

Chronic use leads to a condition called ginsing abuse syndrome that constitutes symptoms such as diarrhea nervousness, insomnia and dermatosis.

Management

Simple withdrawal of the drug leads to disappearance of syndrome.

GLIBENCLAMIDE (Antidiabetic)

It is an oral antidiabetic agent given for treatment of diabetes mellitus.

Symptoms

Hypoglycemia with impariment of consciousness, hypertonia, hyperreflexia, dilated pupils (may or may not be), dryness of skin, cerebral oedema and neurogenic diabetes insipidus.

Management

Activated charcoal is helpful in removing unabsorbed drug. **No purgative is required.**

Hypoglycemia should be corrected urgently. Large amount of intravenous dextrose may not be sufficient to restore normal blood glucose concentrations.

Glycogen has been recommended if the patient presents within 1 or 2 hours of ingestion. **Glycogen is not effective after 24-36 hours of ingestion** because glucose and glycogen will further stimulate insulin release and increase the tendency to produce hypoglycemia.

G

Diazoxide: Administer diazoxide, initial dose is 1-25 mg/kg body weight given over 1 hour and repeated 6 hourly. With diazoxide plasma potassium tends to fall and therefore the patient must be monitored carefully for serum K^+. Diazoxide tends to cause sodium and water retention therefore avoid in patients of hypertension and congestive cardiac failure.

For treatment of convulsions administer diazepam 5-10 mg I/V or phenytoin (10-15 mg/kg I/V) or phenobarbitone (10-12 mg/kg/IV).

Cerebral oedema should be treated conventionally.

When acute phase is over and repeated activated charcoal is not being used, dizoxide may be given orally 5 mg/kg in two or three divided doses daily until there is no risk of hypoglycemia.

Forced diuresis and haemodialysis are ineffective.

GLIBURIDE (Antidiabetic)

An oral hypoglycemic agent 10-15 mg caused profound hypoglycemia while in non-diabetic person even 5 mg caused hypoglycemia.

Clinical Picture and Treatment

Same as with **Glibenclamide** *(Refer page 60)*.

GLYCERYL TRINITRATE (Antianginal)

Glyceryl trinitrate is a widely used vasodilator for the treatment of ischemic heart disease and heart failure.

Symptoms of Toxicity

Headache, flushing of skin and orthostatic hypotension with reflex tachycardia are the adverse effects of nitrates and nitrites that occur commonly. Accidental toxicity in children and intentional poisoning in adults are reported.

Workers or patients regularly exposed to nitrates may develop tolerance and may suffer angina or myocardial infarction owing to rebound coronary vasoconstriction upon sudden withdrawal of this drug.

Management

Maintain patency of airway and assist ventilation if necessary. Administer supplemental oxygen.

G

Vasodilator overdose induced hypotension usually responds to supine positioning. In case no effect is seen, manage as follows:

a. Fluid therapy must be instituted at the rate of 10-20 ml/kg.
b. Dopamine—Infuse 5 μg/kg/min.

Symptomatic methemoglobinemia may be treated with methylene blue. It is indicated if patient has symptoms or signs of hypoxemia (e.g. dyspnea, confusion and chest pain) or methemoglobinemia is over 30%.

Dosage of methylene blue (adults and children): 1-2 mg/kg (0.1-0.2 ml/kg of 1% solution) IV slowly over 5 minutes. May be repeated in 30-60 minutes. If no response occurs, do not repeat dosing. Severe methemoglobinemia in infants not responsive to methylene blue therapy may require exchange transfusion.

Toxicity due to ingestion

Ingestion: Administer activated charcoal if available. Ipecac induced emesis may be useful for initial treatment at the scene. Gastric emptying is not necessary for small ingestion if activated charcoal can be given promptly.

Hemodialysis and hemoperfusion are not effective.

H

HEMLOCK WATER DROPWORT (Plants)

Water hemlock and hemlock water drop are highly poisonous plants. Poisoning usually occurs due to ingestion of the roots.

Symptoms of Toxicity: Appear one hour after ingestion.

Malaise, nausea, hypersalivation, vomiting, abdominal cramps, extensor muscle spasm, opisthotonous, convulsions, dilated pupils, cyanosis, pyrexia, bradycardia, tachycardia, parotid enlargement, flushing of the skin, leukocytosis, metabolic acidosis, elevated aspartate aminotransferase, toxic myositis, jaundice and hypoprothrombinaemia.

Management

No specific treatment is available. The stomach should be emptied by gastric lavage.

Diazepam in usual doses to be given if patient has convulsions.

Dantrolene: (If muscle tone is increased) 1-2 mg/kg IV rapidly may be repeated as needed every 5-10 minutes to a total dose of 10 mg/kg. This is followed by 1-2 mg/kg IV or orally upto maximum 100 mg 4 times a day for 2-3 days to prevent recurrence of hyperthermia.

Other symptoms should be treated symptomatically.

HEPTACHLOR (Organochlorine)

It is widely used as a pesticide in agriculture, insect control and malarial control programmes. It is moderately toxic among organochlorines with animal oral $LD_{50} > 50$ mg/kg.

Symptoms of Toxicity

CNS: Confusion, tremors, obtundation, coma, seizures and respiratory depression.

Sudden onset of convulsions not preceded by the above premonitory manifestations are possible with delayed and recurrent seizures.

CVS: Arrhythmia may occur owing to myocardial sensitivity to catecholamines.

GIT: Nausea, vomiting.

Management

Same as for other **Organochlorines** *(Refer page 218).*

HEROIN (Opioid)

H

It is diacetylmorphine and is 6 times more potent than morphine. It is not used clinically but is one of the favoured drug of abuse.

Clinical Picture and Treatment

Same as for other **Opioids** *(Refer page 215).*

HONEY (Food Item)

Bees can collect nector from poisonous plants and the resultant honey can be toxic. Most common variety of toxic honey is collected from the lourll flowers and rtodendrons.

Symptoms

On ingestion—Vomiting, diarrhea tingling on extremeties and mental disturbances.

Management is symptomatic.

HONEY BEES STING

Honey bee stings when threatened or harmed. These have a barbed stinger which contains 2 lancets which become firmly attached to human skin resulting in dis-engagement of the whole sting apparatus from abdomen resulting in death of the bee. Yet the reflex action of the attached muscles may continue to inject venom for some time.

Bee venom contains histamine, dopamine and certain neurotoxins.

Symptoms

There is local pain with erythema and sometimes oedema. Anaphylactic reaction is common in atopic individuals. Symptoms range from mild urticaria, pruritis and flushing to severe anaphylactic symptomatology (hypotension, laryngeal edema and bronchospasm).

Abdominal pain and diarrhea may also be reported.

Delayed hypersensitive, neurological and renal manifestations may also occur.

Management

Anaphylactic reaction needs immediale attention. Adrenaline I/V (0.1 ml of 1:1000 adrenaline in 10 ml salin) along with oxygen and assisted ventilation are necessary measures.

Anti histamines like diphenhydramine hydrochloride 1.25 mg/kg given I/M or I/V depending upon the situation.

Steroids are recommended only if symptoms of allergy persist. Aminophylline 250 mg I/V is given slowly over a period of 15 minutes to relieve bronchospasm or inhaled salbutamol can be tried. Stinger needs to be scraped off. **Avoid pulling the sting as it squeezes venom sac and inject venom into human.**

Wash sting or bite site with povidone iodine and apply calamine lotion or cold compresses of magnesium sulfate.

HONEYSUCKLE (Plant)

Berries are often eaten by children. If belongs to Lonicera species that contains cyanogenic glycosides, alkaloids and sponins.

Symptoms of Toxicity

Majority of cases are not associated with ill effects but few of them may develop abdominal pain and vomiting.

Treatment

Symptomatic treatment should be followed as there is no specific antidote.

HYDRALAZINE (Vasodilator)

It is a peripheral vasodilator and serious acute overdose seldom occurs. Hypotension with tachycardia are the main symptoms.

Minimum toxic levels have not been established.

Symptoms of Toxicity

Headache, Dizziness, Syncope, Ataxia.

Nausea.
Weakness.
Orthostatic hypotension.
Warm flushed skin.
Palpitation.
Lethargy.

Severe hypotension may result in cerebral and myocardial ischemia and acute renal failure.

Management

H

If the patient is unconscious or drowsy lay him or her on one side in the recovery position. Check breathing every 10 minutes and keep the patient warm.

Assisted ventilation with oxygen supplementation should be provided if it is necessary.

For decontamination, activated charcoal is effective. Gastric emptying is not necessary if activated charcoal is given promptly.

Vasodilator overdose induced hypotension usually responds to supine positioning. In case no effect is seen, manage as follows:

a. Fluid therapy must be instituted at the rate of 10-20 ml/kg.
b. Dopamine. Infuse 2.5-5 μg/kg/min.

HYDROCHLORIC ACID

HCl is present in the digestive juices of the human stomach. Industrially, it is used to process steel, in production of batteries, photoflash bulbs and fireworks. It is used in several other industries like milk, food, paper, pharmaceutical, electronics and chemical technical industry for wastewater treatment, cleaning, neutralization for hydrolysing proteins, and for the removal of lime and oxalate residues.

Clincal Picture

Toxicity due to hydrochloric acid is treated symptomatically in the same manner as hydrofluoric acid *(Refer page 149)*.

HYDROCYANIC ACID

Is also known as Prussic acid. It is colourless gas with penetrating odour and combines with alkalies to produce cyanides. Hydrocyanic acid is liberated when sodium or potassium cyanide interact with hydrochloric acid in the stomach. Liberated hydrocyanic acid readily penetrates gastric mucosa and causes systemic toxicity.

It is also found in vegetable kernels of peaches, almonds and plums in the form of glucoside amygdalin. **Apple seeds contain HCN in good amount.**

Symptoms and Signs

If large amount has been consumed or inhaled death occurs in minutes. It is one of the most rapidly acting poison.

With smaller doses there is dyspnea, convulsions and dilated pupils.

In very small concentrations patient experiences headache, confusion, giddiness and loss of muscular power. Breath smells of bitter almonds. Chronic poisoning occurs from repeated exposures to sublithal doses of acid/salt in photographers. Headache, vomiting, diarrhea, loss of appetite and mental disturbances are common features of chronic poisoning.

Fatal dose is 60 mg of hydrocyanic acid or 60 drops of crude oil of bitter almonds.

Average fatal period with small doses is 20-30 minutes and moderate doses 2-10 minutes.

Management

Amyl nitrite inhalation 0.2 ml ampoule and repeated every 3 minutes or 10 ml of 3% sodium nitrate I/V slowly.

Para amino propiopherone may also help or

Slow I/V infusion of 25% sodium thiosulphate.

Stomach lavage with 5-10% sodium thiosulphate followed by potassium carbonate is recommended.

Circulatory and respiratory back ups are required. Survival for 4 hours is followed by recovery.

HYDROFLUORIC ACID

Hydrofluoric acid is used in the purification of aluminum, uranium, stainless steel and silicon. It is also used in the synthesis of fluorine containing organic compounds.

Symptoms

In case of ingestion:

GIT: Severe burning pain in the mouth, throat, abdomen, dysphagia, gastritis, vomiting, diarrhoea (bloody, mucoid).

CVS: Hypotension with cold clammy skin and rapid pulse.

Miscellaneous: Metabolic acidosis, hemolysis, massive fluid and electrolyte shifts (hyperkalemia, hyperphosphatemia, hypocalcemia, hyperchloremia).

In case of inhalation: Cough, dyspnea, pleuritic chest pain, pulmonary oedema, frothy sputum, hemoptysis, bronchospasm, pain in eyes and lacrimation.

In case of eye exposure: Irritation, pain, lacrimation, swelling, chemosis, photophobia, corneal erosion and perforation, necrosis of conjunctiva and cornea.

In case of dermal exposure: Burning pain, irritation, redness, blistering ulceration.

Management

In case of Ingestion:

Do not induce vomiting.

Administer water or milk to dilute acid.

In case of inhalation: Patient should be shifted to fresh air.

In case of eye exposure: irrigate with large volumes of 0.9% normal saline or water for 15 minutes or more depending upon the severity.

Eyes should not be washed with soap solution.

Wash affected skin with copious amounts of water or mild soap solution.

Do not give gastric lavage.

Endotracheal intubation to be done in case of airway compromise.

100% humidified oxygen given with assisted ventilation.

Suction should be done by soft nasogastric tube.

Irrigate mouth with water in a cooperative patient and intubate unconscious patients.

IV fluids given: Volume to be determined by the condition of the patient.

Vasopressors to be given if needed.

Give antibiotics to prevent infections.

Perform endoscopy within first 24 hours and chest X-ray for detection of mediastinitis or GI perforation.

Perform laparotomy in case endoscopy reveals grade, necrosis of oesophagus or stomach or if features of GI perforation are evident at the time of admission.

For burns on skin/mouth wash immediately with water for atleast 15 min.

In case of HF poisoning monitor ECG, serum Ca^{++}. If there is evidence of hypocalcemia or severe hypokalemia give calcium gluconate (10%) 2-4 ml/kg IV.

For topical exposure apply gel containing calcium gluconate (2.5 g/100 ml lubricant).

Do not give excessive amount of milk or water as this provokes vomiting.

Do not give carbonated beverages or bicarbonate for neutralization.

H

HYDROGEN PEROXIDE

Hydrogen peroxide is a strong oxidizing agent and rapidly breaks into oxygen and water. Generation of oxygen gas in closed body cavities causes mechanical distension resulting in gastric/intestinal perforation.

In case of ingestion: Burns on lips, oral mucosa, upper airway and oesophagus. Drooling strider vomiting and gastrointestinal bleeding.

In case of inhalation: Upper airway oedema, dyspnea, wheezing, pulmonary oedema, pneumonitis and respiratory failure.

In case of eye exposure: Conjunctival irritation, chemosis, corneal perforation, distortion of cellular membranes, loss of cornea, conjunctival and lens epithelium and loss of endothelium of cornea and blood vessels.

In case of skin exposure: Pain, redness, irritation with full thickness burns.

Management

In case of ingestion:

Do not induce vomiting but administer water or milk. Do not perform gastric lavage.

In case of inhalation: Patient should be shifted to fresh air.

In case of eye exposure: Irrigate eyes with large volumes of 0.9% normal saline or water for 15 minutes or more depending upon severity of burns.

Eyes should not be washed with soap solution.

Wash affected skin with copious amounts of water or mild soap solution.

Perform endotracheal intubation in case of airway compromise.

Administer 100% humidified oxygen with assisted ventilation.

Suction should be done by soft nasogastric tube.

Irrigate mouth with water in cooperative patient or intubate unconscious patients.

Administer IV fluids according to the need of the patient.

Vasopressors to be given if required.

Antibiotics are given to prevent infections.

H

Perform endoscopy within first 24 hours and chest X-ray for mediastinitis or GI perforation.

Perform laprotomy if endoscopy reveals necrosis of oesophagus or stomach or if clinical features are suggestive of GI perforation at the time of initial presentation.

Activated charcoal is not effective.

HYDROGEN SULFIDE

It is a highly toxic, flammable, colourless gas that is heavier than air. It is produced naturally by decaying organic matter and is also a by-product of many industrial processes. High levels are likely to be found in petroleum refineries, tanneries, mines, pulp-making factories, sulfur hot springs, carbon disulfide production, hot asphalt fumes and pools of sewage sulfide or liquid menure. **'Stink Bombs'** contain hydrogen sulfide that may occassionally cause accidental poisoning of large group. **Though hydrogen sulfide has strong unpleasant small paradoxically its smell cannot be perceived if its concentration is too high.** This is due to paralysis of olfactory nerves leading to serious toxicity.

Symptoms of Toxicity

Acute symptoms include headache, nausea and vomiting, dizziness, confusion, seizures and coma. Massive exposure may cause immediate cardiovascular collapse, respiratory arrest and death.

At low levels upper airway irritation, burning eyes and blepharospasm may occur. Skin exposure can cause immediate cardiovascular collapse, respiratory arrest and death.

Management

Rescuers should use breathing apparatus to prevent personal exposure.

Remove the victim from site of exposure and give supplemental oxygen.

Maintain the airway and assist ventilation if necessary. Administer highly humidified supplemental oxygen.

Treat coma, seizures and hypotension by standard methods.

No specific antidote is available. However, administration of **nitrites** to produce methemoglobinemia may promote conversion of sulfide ion to sulphenoglobin which is far less toxic.

There is no role for enhanced elimination procedures such as dialysis or dialysis or hemoperfusion.

HYDROMORPHONE (Opioid)

It is an opioid used in treatment of moderate to severe pain.

Clinical Picture and Treatment

Same as for other **Opioids** *(Refer page 215).*

HYMENOPTERA (Animal toxin)

Most bees sting only when disturbed but yellow jackets attack without provocation. These are the most common cause of insect induced anaphylactic reactions.

Symptoms

Once the venom is injected, there is immediate onset of severe pain followed by local inflammatory reaction (erythema, wheal formation, ecchymosis, edema, vesiculation and blisters, itching and a sensation of warmth). Multiple stings also produce vomiting, diarrhoea, hypotension, syncope, cyanosis, dyspnea, rhabdomyolysis, coagulopathy and death.

Most anaphylactic reactions occur within 15 minutes of envenomation. Sometimes, delayed onset reactions may occur including arthritis (arthralgias, fever), nephritis, transverse myelitis and Guillain-Barre syndrome.

Management

Monitor the victim closely for at least 30-60 minutes.

Treat anaphylaxis, with **epinephrine and diphenhydramine.** Persistent urticaria may respond to the addition of cimetidine, 300 mg orally or IV. **Persons known**

to be sensitive to Hymenoptera venom should carry epinephrine emergency kit at all times.

Provide tetanus prophylaxis if the patient is not already immunized.

There is no available antidote.

Examine the sting site carefully for any retained stingers. These can be removed by gentle scraping with a knife blade.

Wash the area with soap and water.

H

HYPOGLYCEMIC AGENTS (Sulphonylureas and Insulin)

Agents used to lower blood glucose are divided into two groups, the oral hypoglycemics and insulin products. The oral hypoglycemic agents are sulfonylureas and all these agents vary in onset and duration of blood glucose lowering effects.

Symptoms

Management

IPECAC induced emesis may be useful for initial treatment provided it can be given within a few minutes of exposure. Gastric emptying is not necessary if activated charcoal with purgative can be given promptly.

Maintain airway and assist ventilation if necessary.

Treat coma and seizures by appropriate drugs if these occur.

Administer concentrated glucose intravenously (dextrose 25%).

Follow serum glucose levels closely for several hours after the last dose of dextrose. Give repeated boluses of glucose.

For patients with oral hypoglycemic overdose, consider intravenous diazoxide.

For treatment of Insulin induced hypoglycemia

Orally ingested insulin is not absorbed and produces no toxicity. So gut decontamination is not necessary.

Alkalization of the urine increases renal elimination of insulin. **Dialysis procedures are of no value for either insulin or oral hypoglycemic agents.**

Administer potassium chloride with constant monitoring of serum K^+.

For details see **Insulin (Hormone)** *(Refer page 60).*

I

IBUPROFEN (NSAID)

It is one of the most widely used drug for anti-inflammatory activity. It is rapidly absorbed from the gut, extensively metabolized and eliminated therefore half life is short (3 hours).

Symptoms of Toxicity

Ingestion of less than 100 mg/kg body usually does not result in toxic symptoms but more than 400 mg/kg can cause serious toxicity and features associated with it.

Drowsiness, vomiting, abdominal discomfort, tinnitus, blurred vision and tachycardia are the common symptoms of toxicity. Other serious complications are **coma, convulsions, apnea and bradycardia.**

Abnormalities in liver and renal function test may be seen.

Management

Only those patients require treatment who show toxic symptoms.

Repeated doses of activated charcoal should be given (30-100 gm of charcoal).

Treatment should be supportive and care should be taken to maintain a patent airway.

Since plasma half life of ibuprofen is short, **Elimination techniques are irrelevant.** Maintaining BP and kidney functions help recovery.

IMIPRAMINE (Antidepressant)

It is a tricyclic antidepressant and is used in the treatment of depression.

Symptoms of Toxicity

Mild: Confusion, blurred vision, flushed dry skin and mucosa, sinus tachycardia and hypotension.

Moderate to severe: Mydrasis, agitation, visual and auditory hallucinations, myoclonus, convulsions, ataxia, coma, hypotension, sinus tachycardia and other brady-arrhythmias with prolonged PR and QRS duration (100 m sec) metabolic acidosis, respiratory insufficiency or arrest, pulmonary edema, oesophageal spasm and urinary retention.

Death is due to cardiac arrest and circulatory failure.

Management

Induce emesis by mechanical stimulation of the back of the tongue.

Place a spoon in patient's mouth in case of seizures to prevent injury to tongue.

Maintain proper airway and ensure adequate oxygenation.

Nasopharyngeal suction to be done.

Catheterise if patient has urinary retention. This is indicated if bladder is full.

Gastric Lavage

Activated charcoal to be used initially with purgative. Repeat doses should not contain purgative

For controlling seizures use **diazepam** in usual doses I.V.

Repeat every 10-15 min.

Or

Lorazepam: 1-2 mg IV given over several minutes.

IV fluids are administered: According to the need of the patient.

Sodium bicarbonate: 500-800 ml IV slow infusion (7.5%v.v.) to maintain a blood pH of 7.5.

Dobutamine: 2.5-1.5 μg/kg/min infusion, if hypotension is present.

Potassium chloride: To be given only if serum K^+ is low and with monitoring.

Special Precautions to be Taken

Avoid antiarrhythmic drugs like quinidine and procainamide as they decrease AV nodal conduction.

Do not give phenothiazines for treating hyperthermia as their own anticholinergic action adds to that of the poison.

As far as possible avoid dopamine to treat hypotension as its adrenergic effect increases arrythmogenicity. If necessary use low doses.

Treat seizures immediately so as to prevent hypoxia and lactic acidosis which may predispose to development of ventricular arrhythmia.

Use of phenytoin for seizure should be avoided as it increases incidence of ventricular tachycardia.

Avoid propranolol and verapamil as they slow conduction velocity and heart rate and lower BP.

Patients with history of unconsciousness should be observed for 24 hours after recovery.

Potassium replacement with bicarbonate should be done cautiously as hyperkalemia may aggravate imprамine induced cardiac arrhythmias.

INDORAMIN (Antihistaminic, Antiadrenergic)

It is selective α_1-adrenoreceptor blocker and competitive antagonist of histamine H_1 and 5 HT receptors. It is a peripheral vasodilator used in treatment of hypertension and serious acute overdoses seldom occur.

Minimum toxic level has not been established.

Symptoms of Toxicity

Headache, nausea, dizziness, weakness, syncope, orthostatic hypotension, warm flushed skin, palpitation, lethargy and ataxia.

Severe hypotension may result in cerebral and myocardial ischemia and acute renal failure.

Management

If the patient is unconscious or drowsy lay him or her on one side in the recovery position. Check breathing every 10 minutes and keep the patient warm.

Assisted ventilation with oxygen supplementation should be provided if necessary.

For decontamination, activated charcoal is effective. Gastric emptying is not necessary if activated charcoal is given promptly.

Hypotension due to this drug responds to supine positioning of the patient. In case no effect is seen, manage as described below:

a. IV Fluid therapy must be instituted at the rate of 10-20 ml/kg.
b. Dopamine. Infuse 5-10 μg/kg/min overdose in severe peripheral vasoconstriction and gangrene.

INSULIN (Hormone)

It is the most commonly used hormone in patients with insulin dependent diabetes mellitus.

Symptoms of Toxicity

Examination will reveal the usual signs and symptoms of hypoglycemia and other associated complications like cerebral oedema and brain damage.

Hypoglycemia in a diabetic is common in labile diabetics. It can also occur due to high dose or missing a meal or by performing strenuous exercise.

Symptoms of Hypoglycemia

Symptoms of hypoglycemia differ from individual to individual usually sympathetic symptoms occur initially followed by CNS symptoms. **Over a period of time 30% of diabetic patients do not exhibit sympathetic symptoms.**

Sympathetic stimulation—sweating, palpitations, tremors.

CNS—Dizziness, headache, visual disturbances, and behavioural changes.

Miscellaneous: Fatigue and weakness and fall in BP may sometimes be seen.

Management

If the clinical signs of hypoglycemia are evident, the blood glucose should be measured to corroborate the diagnosis.

To counteract the hypoglycemia administer 50 ml of 50% of glucose intravenously. Then give a 10% of dextrose infusion.

As soon as the patient is fit to eat, give a carbohydrate rich diet.

Cerebral oedema should be treated by hyperventilation of the patient till the P_aCO_2 lies between 3.0 and 3.4 KPa. Although this treatment is recommended the poisoning is complicated by coexisting severe hypotension.

Mannitol 1g/kg body weight (20%) should be given intravenously.

Dextramethasone intramuscularly is recommended for long term management but may not be effective in patients with generalised brain oedema.

IODINE (Tincture Iodine, Mandle's Throat Paint)

Iodine is commonly used as an antiseptic and germicide agent. Also, used in dyes and X-ray media.

Symptoms of Toxicity

In case of ingestion: Burns on lips, oral mucosa, in air passages, oesophagus, strider, vomiting and gastrointestinal bleeding.

In case of inhalation: Upper airway oedema, dyspnoea, wheezing, pulmonary oedema, pneumonitis, strider, followed by respiratory failure.

In case of eye exposure: Conjunctival irritation, chemosis, corneal, perforation, or distortion of cellular membranes, loss of corneal conjunctival and lens epithelium and loss of endothelium of cornea and blood vessels.

In case of skin exposure: Pain, redness, irritation, and deep burns.

Management

In case of inhalation: Patient should be shifted to fresh air.

In case of eye exposure: Irrigate with large volumes of 0.9% normal saline or water for 15 minutes or more depending upon severity.

Wash affected skin with copious amounts of water or mild soap solution.

In case of Ingestion:

Do not induce vomiting.

Administer milk or water immediately to dilute iodine.

Do not give gastric lavage.

Do endotracheal intubation in case of airway compromise.

Administer 100% humidified oxygen with assisted ventilation.

Suction should be done by soft nasogastric tube.

Irrigate mouth with water in cooperative patients or intubate unconscious patients.

Give IV fluids, according to the need of the patient.

Give vasopressors, if necessary.

Perform endoscopy within first 24 hours and chest X-ray for mediastinitis or GI perforation.

I

Perform laparotomy if endoscopy reveals necrosis of oesophagus or stomach or if signs and symptoms of GI perforation are obvious at the time of admission.

Role of enhanced elimination: Once absorbed into the circulation, iodine is rapidly converted to the far less toxic iodide. **Therefore there is no need for enhanced drug removal.**

I

IODOFENPHOS (Organophosphorus Compound)

It belongs to organophosphorus group of widely used pesticides that may cause acute or chronic poisoning. It is a relatively less toxic organophosphorus compound with an LD_{50} of 2100 mg/kg.

Symptoms and Management

Same as of other **Organophosphorus compounds** *(Refer page 219)*.

IRON (Hematinic)

It is a commonly used hematinic, available as over the counter preparation.Therefore, it remains one of the most common cause of childood toxicity and the leading cause of fatal poisonings in children.

Toxic dose: Most pediatric iron formulations contain 12-18 mg of elemental iron per dose while most adult preparations contain 60-80 mg of elemental iron per dose. The fatal amount of elemental iron is estimated to be between 180 and 300 mg/kg body weight. Serious toxicity occurs when 60 mg or more elemental iron /kg bodyweight has been ingested.

Toxic Serum Iron Levels

Mild toxicity >450-500 μg/dl.

Severe toxicity >800-1000 μg/dl.

Total iron-binding capacity is not reliable in iron overdose and should not be used to estimate free iron levels.

Symptoms of Toxicity

Most of the toxic effects are due to hemorrhagic necrosis in GIT often leading to perforation. Absorbed iron causes cellular dysfunction resulting in lactic acidosis and necrosis. **Clinical course runs in 4 phases:**

First Phase (Occurs within first few hours after ingestion)

It is characterized by vomiting, diarrhoea and abdominal pain. The vomitus and stools are usually dark grey or black in colour (due to iron). They may also be blood stained due to corrosive effects on the upper gastrointestinal mucosa.

Most cases of mild poisoning do not go beyond this phase.

However in case of severe poisoning, drowsiness, coma, convulsions, metabolic acidosis and shock can occur.

Mostly there is no mortality at this stage, but a few can die due to progressive circulatory failure and coma.

Second Phase (Occurs 6-12 hours after ingestion)

During this phase, symptoms subside as iron is taken up by the reticulo endothetial system.

Third Phase (Occurs 12-48 hours after ingestion)

A few patients may suffer this phase. This phase is characterized by severe shock, metabolic acidosis, jaundice, coagulation abnormalities, hypoglycemia and renal failure. **This phase has high mortality.**

Fourth Phase (2-5 weeks after ingestion)

Occurs in patients who survive after third phase.

Symptoms are due to formation of gastric strictures and pyloric stenosis (alone or in combination) and is characterised by obstructive symptoms.

Diagnosis is based on

History of exposure.

Presence of vomiting, diarrhoea, hypotension and other clinical signs.

WBC > 15,000 or blood glucose >150 mg/dl or visible radiopaque pills in abdominal X-ray.

Management

Induce emesis with Ipecac. It should be instituted early (before bringing the patient to hospital) as it is not effective if given late. **Activated charcoal is not effective.**

Maintain patent airway and provide assisted ventilation if necessary.

Gastric lavage should be done as quickly as possible. **Do not use phosphate solutions for lavage as this may result**

in hypernatremia, hyperphosphatemia and hypocalcemia.

Do not add deferoxamine to the lavage fluid as it increases iron absorption.

It is advisable to repeat abdomen X-ray. Perform whole bowel irrigation if X-ray shows presence of radiopaque pills in the GIT after gastric lavage.

Blood replacement and intravenous crystalloid fluids are needed to correct hypovolemic shock.

I

For treatment of convulsions: Use Diazepam in undiluted form. Closely monitor blood pressure and respiration.

Administer sodium bicarbonate for treating metabolic acidosis.

Deferoxamine is the specific antidote for iron poisoning. Its administration results in characteristic orange or pink red (Vin rose) colour of urine (which is due to the formation of chelated deferoxamine-iron complex). **Terminate chelator therapy once the colour of the urine turns normal.**

Intravenous Dose: 10-15 mg/kg/hr given by constant infusion. **(Higher infusion rate may cause hypotension).** Maximum dose is 6 gm/day.

Intramuscular Dose: This route is used for the administration of test dose. The dose is 50 mg/kg with a maximum of 1 gm. Hypotension can occur with this route also.

Hemodilaysis and hemoperfusion are ineffective but may be of importance in patients of renal failure.

ISOCARBOXAZID (Antidepressant MAO Inhibitor)

It is used as an antidepressant and serious toxicity results from overdose or due to interactions with certain other drugs or foods.

Toxic Dose

Ingestion of even 2-3 mg/kg of the drug may be life threatening. As it causes irreversible inhibition of the enzyme (MAO), adverse drug interactions may occur for upto 2 weeks after discontinuing them.

Signs and Symptoms of Toxicity

Even after acute ingestion of the overdose of isocarboxazid, it takes 6-24 hours before symptoms are evident. However, if interacting drug/food is taken in the meantime, toxicity may be precipitated immediately.

Mild Toxicity

Anxiety.
Flushing.
Headache.
Tremors.
Myoclonus.
Hyperreflexia.
Sweating.
Shivering.
Tachypnea.
Moderate degree of hypertension.
Orthostatic hypotension is also a possibility.

Severe Toxicity

Severe hypertension may result in intracranial hemorrhage

Delirium

Hyperthermia

Cardiovascular collapse and multisystem failure are the causes of death.

Serotonin Syndrome

This syndrome occurs when patients poisoned with MAO inhibitor consumes one of the following drugs/foods; meperidine, dextromethorphan, fluoxetine, paroxetine, sertraline or tryptophan. It is characterized by severe rigidity, hyperthermia myoclonic jerking hyperreflexia and diaphoresis.

Management

Maintenance of airway and ventilation is important. If deemed necessary, assisted ventilation with oxygen supplementation may be provided.

Treat hypertension by the use of any one of the following drugs:

Phentolamine: 1-5 mg IV (children 0.02-0.1 mg/kg) as a bolus. Repeat at 5-10 minutes intervals (or constant infusion of 0.1-2 mg/min) as needed to lower blood pressure to a desired level (usually <100 mg/Hg diastolic in adults and 80 mm Hg diastolic in children).

Or

Nifedipine: 10 mg sublingually for adults and 0.25-0.5 mg/kg/dose for children. **Do not use extended release formulation for sublingual administration.**

Or

Nitroprusside: It should only be used in emergency or intensive care setting. Blood pressure should be monitored continuously or frequently.

Dosage: For preparation of the intravenous solution, dissolve 50 mg of sodium nitroprusside in 3 ml of 5% dextrose and dilute this solution in 5% dextrose to achieve a concentration of 200, 100 or 50 µg/ml, respectively. Initiate with 0.3 µg/kg/min and titrate the dose to a desired effect. In case no effect on blood pressure is seen, use an alternative.

The average dose is 3 µg/kg/min in children and adults. Maximum rate should not exceed 10 µg/kg/min to avoid risk of acute cyanide toxicity.

Nitroprusside solution is photosensitive therefore, the bottle and intravenous tubing should be protected from light.

In case, tachycardia is also present, add one of the following to the above mentioned treatment.

Propranolol: 0.02-0.1 mg/kg IV.

Esmolol: 25-100 µg/kg/min IV.

Labetolol: 0.2-0.3 mg/kg IV.

Do not use beta blockers alone for treatment of hypertension as it results in paradoxical rise in BP specially when rise in BP is caused primarily by alpha-stimulation.

In case of abnormal neurological findings, a CT scan is advisable to rule out stroke.

Convulsions should be managed by described below:

Diazepam: Diazepam should be given in undiluted form and closely monitor blood pressure and respiration.

Followed by:

Phenytoin:

Or

Phenobarbitone

For treating serotonin syndrome, use diazepam for controlling seizures as described above and apply external cooling.

Treat hyperthermia by external cooling. This evaporative method is the most efficient way of cooling. In case shivering occurs as a consequence of cooling, use diazepam (0.1-0.2 mg/kg IV) or midazolam (0.05-0.1 mg/kg IV) to prevent or treat it.

Continuously monitor body temperature, vital signs and ECG for a minimum of 6 hours in asymptomatic and admit all symptomatic patients.

ISONIAZID (Antitubercular drug) (INH)

It is used as a first line drug to treat tuberculosis.

Isoniazid is acetylated and individuals may be slow or fast acetylators. Hence, toxicity of INH depends on genetic trait.

The toxicity of isoniazid may be precipitated due to acute pyridoxine deficiency and reduction in brain concentration of GABA.

Symptoms

Within 2-4 hours of ingestion, commonly encountered symptoms are nausea, vomiting and hallucinations.

There is a possibility of aspiration pneumonia and respiratory failure. Severe metabolic acidosis, raised serum lactate concentrations, hypoxia, hyperpyrexia, rhabdomylosis and acute renal failure may be seen.

Hypoglycemia, polymorph leukocytosis, elevation of serum osmolality, aspartate aminotransferase and lactate dehydrogenase have also been seen.

Plasma INH concentrations rarely exceed 150 ng/L, although values upto 250 ng/16 hours after ingestion have been reported.

Management

Establish and maintain a patent airway.

Gastric emptying and supportive therapy is done for mild form of poisoning.

Pyridoxine

5 g pyridoxine is given IV slowly over 30-60 minutes and repeated if convulsions are not controlled.

Repeated activated charcoal should be given after stabilization of the patient.

Methods aimed at increasing the elimination of the drugs from body forced diuresis are not beneficial. In case of very serious patients **haemoperfusion has been recommended.**

ISOPROPANOL (Alcohol)

It is isopropyl alcohol used in disinfectants, windscreen washes cosmetics and pharmaceutical preparatory meant for external use. It is infected/abused by alcoholics. It is metabolised by alcohol dehydrase.

Symptoms

Features resemble those of ethanol poisoning with loss of consciousness, hypotension, hyporeflexia, vasodilation, respiratory depression and hypothermia but the characteristic odour of ethanol is absent.

There is increased mortality among severely hypotensive patients.

In general the depressant effects of isopropanol are twice that of ethanol and the incidence of nausea, vomiting and abdominal pain are more common with ethanol.

Other rare complications (in severe intoxication) are possible renal failure, rhabdomylosis, myoglobinuria, hemolytic anemia and elevation of CSF protein content.

Management

Gastric emptying and supportive therapy is done for mild form of poisoning.

For those who have a high isopropanol concentration of greater than 4 g/l require hemodialysis for removal of isopropanol and its metabolites from the blood.

ISOXATHION (Organophosphorus)

It belongs to organophosphorus group of widely used pesticides that may cause acute or chronic poisoning. It is a moderately toxic organophosphorus compound with an LD_{50} of 180-242 mg/kg.

Clinical Picture and Management

Same as with other **Organophosphorus compounds** *(Refer page 219)*.

J

JELLY FISH (Animal Toxin)

It belongs to phylus Cnidaria that also includes fire coral, Portuguese man-of-war, Box Jelly fish, sea wasps, sea nettle and anemones. Microscopic structures called nematocysts on the surface of jelly fish contain venom.

Symptoms

Local reactions: Immediate in onset, burning pain and pruritic rash appear. Papular lesions appear leading to pustules and desquamation followed by **systemic effects** such as paresthesias, anaphylactic symptoms, hypotension, muscle spasm, local edema and hemolysis.

Chills, fever, nausea, vomiting, abdominal pain, myalgias, arthralgias, ataxia, paralysis, coma, seizures and cardiac arrhythmias.

Box jelly fish envenomation is associated with rapid onset of cardiovascular collapse which may give rise to lethal outcomes.

Management

Maintain airway and assist ventilation if necessary. Administer supplemental oxygen.

Treat convulsions if they occur initially by diazepam followed by either phenytoin or phenobarbitone.

Hypotension is a potential complication of jelly fish poisoning and may be the cause of cardiac arrhythmias.

Fluid therapy must be instituted at the rate of 10-20 ml/kg.

Dopamine. Infuse 5-10 µg/kg/min. Overdose may result in severe peripheral vasoconstriction and gangrene.

Arrhythmias are managed conventionally.

Avoid scratching, scraping or any other mechanical measures that may break open the nematocysts.

Use gloves to wash the affected areas with cold salt water.

Do not use fresh water to wash affected areas because it will cause nematocysts to discharge poison.

The tentacles should be carefully removed with forceps followed by shaving of the affected area to remove the undischarged nematocysts.

For disarming nematocysts, spray, soak or wash the affected area with vinegar for 30 minutes.

Avoid vinegar for treating *Chrysaora quinquecirrha* (American Sea Nettle), *Pelagia noctiloca* and *Cyanea captilata* as vinegar precipitates firing in these species. Application of baking soda for 10 minutes is a good alternative.

JEWELLERY CLEANERS (Mixture of Acids)

In case of ingestion:

Symptoms

Local effects: Burns on lips, oral mucosa, upper airway, oesophagus.

GIT: Drooling strider, vomiting and gastrointestinal bleeding.

In case of inhalation:

Oedema of upper respiratory tract producing dyspnea, wheezing and pulmonary oedema, pneumonitis, respiratory failure.

Exposure of eyes: Conjunctival irritation, corneal perforation, distortion of cellular membranes, loss of epithelium of cornea, conjunctiva and lens.

Skin exposure: Pain, redness, irritation, full thickness burns.

Management

In case of Ingestion:

Avoid inducing vomiting.
Administer water or milk so that acid can be diluted.

Avoid gastric lavage.
In case of airway compromise do endotracheal intubation.

Give 100% humified oxygen for inhalation. Use respirator if available and if deemed necessary.

Suction should be done using soft nasogastric tube.

Irrigate mouth frequently in patients who are cooperative and conscious.

Administer IV fluids—the volume should be determined according to the condition of the patient.

Vasopressors can be used if necessary.

Endoscopy should be performed within first 24 hours to detect presence of perforation.

Perform chest X-ray for detection of mediastinitis or GI perforation. Administer antibiotics if there is mediastinitis perforation.

Laparotomy should be done in case endoscopy reveals necrosis of oesophagus or stomach or when signs and symptoms of GI perforation are evident at the time of initial presentation.

In case of inhalation: Patient should be removed from site of exposure and shifted to fresh air.

In case of eye exposure: Depending upon severity, irrigate with large volumes of 0.9% normal saline or water for 15 minutes or more.

Remove contact lenses.

Wash affected skin with copious amounts of water or mild soap solution.

JODENPHOS (Organophosphorus compound)

It belongs to organophosphorus group of widely used pesticides that may cause acute or chronic poisoning. It is a relatively less toxic organophosphorus compound with an LD_{50} of 2100 mg/kg.

Clinical Picture and Management

Same as with other **Organophosphorus compounds** *(Refer page 219)*.

K

KEPONE (Organochlorine)

It is widely used as a pesticide in agriculture, insect control and malarial control programmes. It is moderately toxic among organochlorines with animal oral $LD_{50} > 50$ mg/kg.

Symptoms of Toxicity

Nausea, vomiting, contusion, tremors, obtundation, coma, seizures and respiratory depression.

Sudden onset of convulsions not preceded by the premonitory manifestations are a possibility (delayed and recurrent seizures).

Arrhythmia may occur owing to myocardial sensitivity to catecholamines.

Management

Move the patient away from contaminated zone.

The clothing should be removed and the whole body should either be sponged or washed with water and soap.

If seizures are present, place a spoon in the mouth of the patient to prevent injury to tongue.

Do not give oil/milk/cream orally.

Emesis is indicated only if patient approaches within 30 minutes of ingestion of organochlorine.

Gastric lavage is advisable if activated charcoal is not available.

Ensure adequate oxygenation and undertake nasopharyngeal suction if necessary.

Give ventilatory support if required.

IV fluids should be given if required—the volume to be determined by the condition of the patient.

For management of seizures administer diazepam in undiluted form and monitor blood pressure. This followed by either Phenytoin or Phenobarbitone for long term control.

Cholestyramine: 4 gms orally is given mixed in fruit juice every 6 hours before meals.

Avoid epinephrine and atropine as these may cause to cardiac arrhythmias.

KEROSENE (Petroleum Product)

Kerosene is an aliphatic hydrocarbon. Accidental poisoning is common in children.

Symptoms of Poisoning

Vomiting is common but not a necessary feature of poisoning. **Diarrhoea is uncommon.**

There may be excitement, but in severe poisoning drowsiness is seen which may lead to coma.

The most common complication of this poisoning is pulmonary troubles which occur in almost 60% of the cases and result from aspiration of kerosene into bronchial tree. This results into cough, choking, wheezing and breathlessness.

Clinical evidence of respiratory involvement is usually evident within few minutes after poisoning but in some cases it may be delayed for hours but not more than a day. Severe poisoning can cause hemorrhagic pulmonary oedema which is fatal within 24 hours. Pneumonitis in most cases involves two or more lobes. Fever and polymorph leukocytosis are common.

Rare complications include pneumatocele formation, intravascular hemolysis and renal failure.

Diagnosis is confirmed by presence of a double gastric level on the X-ray of the abdomen taken in erect position.

Management

Gastric emptying is favoured only if sufficiently large amount has been ingested provided patient should be sufficiently alert so that he can cough effectively and airway should be protected by cuffed endotracheal tube.

Antibiotics should be given in only those patients who develop secondary bacterial infections.

If cyanosis is present, oxygen may be necessary. Intermittant positive pressure is indicated for patients with pulmonary oedema.

Other clinical features are managed symptomatically.

K

L

LABETOLOL (Alpha and Beta Adrenergic Blocker)

It has both alpha and beta adrenoreceptor blocking activity. The alpha blocking activity is 1/10 of phenotolamine and beta blocking potency is 1/3 of propranolol. In large doses it prevents reuptake of catecholamines in adrenergic neurons. It is used to treat pheochromocytoma and to treat rebound hypertension after abrupt withdrawal of clonidine.

Symptoms

In high doses the effects are similar to combination of propranolol and phenoxybenzamine.

Both cardiac output and total peripheral resistance are reduced causing severe fall in BP but heart rate remains unchanged. In contrast to propranolol circulation to limbs increases, thereby making them warm and flushed. **It causes liver damage.**

Management

Raise the foot end of the bed and give I/V fluids.

Administer dopamine to raise blood pressure.

Monitor liver function tests.

Serious toxicity needs symptomatic treatment.

LABURNUM (Plant)

Laburnum anagroides is common plant poison. All parts of the plant specially the bark and seeds are poisonous and it is usually the latter that are involved in childhood poisoning. The main toxic constituent of the laburnum is cytosine.

Symptoms

Nausea, vomiting, increased salivation, drowsiness, incoordination, muscle twitching and convulsions Mydriasis and Tachycardia.

Management

Stomach should be emptied only if a large number of seeds has been ingested. Mild cases do not need treatment.

LACRIMATORS (Tear Gases)

These are aerosol-dispersed chemicals used to control riots.

Chloracetaphenone (CN) methyl chloroform chloro acetaphenone (MACE), chlorobenzylidene-melanonitrile (CS) and dibenzoxazepine (CR) are used for this purpose.

Less often ethyl iodoacetate (KSK) bromobenzyl cyanide (BBC), diphenyl chlorarsine (DA) and dysphenylamine chlorarsine (DM) are also used.

Lacrimators are strong irritators of mucus membranes.

Signs and Symptoms

Eyes: Blepharospasm pain, lacrymation, redness of the conjunctive, periorbital edema. In severe cases there may be corneal edema, keratitis and iridocyclitis.

Respiratory system: Rhinorrhea, cough, sore throat, sneezing etc.

In severe cases there may be acute laryngotracheo bronchitis.

Skin: Erythema, allergic dermatitis and second degree burns may occur. **In severe toxicity fatalities are rare but reported with chloroacetophenone.**

Management

Remove individual from area of contamination. Administer oxygen and give assisted ventilation.

Aminophylline I/V or salbutamol will be needed if patient develops bronchospasm. Wash skin and eyes with plain cold water.

LATHYRUS SATIVU (Kesari Dal)

Peas from this plant are used to adulterate pulses. Prolonged consumption can give rise to lathyrism which is due to a neurotoxin-beta N oxalyl amino-L-alanine.

Symptoms

There is gradual development of spastic paraplegia.

L

Management

Withdrawal of kesari dal from diet and supportive measures.

LEAD

Lead is a very poisonous substance. Lead is used in storage batteries, solder electric cable insulations, paints, pottery and ceramic glazes.

Lead is also used in water supply pipes, in house paints and in pottery which may be used for eating, drinking or cooking. In India it is used as cattle poison and atmosphere lead comes from exhaust pipes of vehicles.

L

Acute exposure rarely causes poisoning but repeated exposures can result in chronic toxicity.

People are at greater risk if atmosphere contains lead dust or fumes. Such as lead smelting, refining, lead battery making, welding and heat stripping of lead paints.

There is a danger of swallowing lead in people who drink or smoke in areas where there are lead fumes or dust.

People may also be poisoned by eating and drinking from lead glazed pottery.

In India lead toxicity is common in chlidren eating mud (picca).

Signs and Symptoms

If breathed in: Following symptoms occur within 24 hours:
Irritation and watering of eyes.
Coughing, choking.
Tightness in chest.
Nausea, vomiting, retching.

After 24 hours:
Rapid, shallow breathing.
Painful cough.
Frothy white or yellowish sputum.
Low blood pressure.

Symptoms after chronic exposure:
Fast pulse. Wrist drop or foot drop, severe anaemia.
Blue line on the gums, colicky pain.
Personality changes, poor memory and slow reactions.
Difficulty in coordinating movement, kidney failure.
Gonadal dysfunction.

Lead from petrol:
Insomnia.
Mental disturbances.
Hallucinations.
Fits.

Management

If the patient is unconscious or drowsy, lay him or her on one side in the recovery position. Check breathing every 10 minutes and keep the patient warm.

General measures: Remove patient from contaminated environment.

Administer purgative like magnesium sulfate.

I/V calcium gluconate (20 ml of 10%) or 10 ml of 5% calcium chloride is given.

Calcium disodium versenate 1 gm diluted in 200-300 ml saline or glucose solution is given. I/V over one hour twice daily for 3-5 days depending on the severity.

A second course is repeated after 5-7 days.

Penicilamine (0.3 to 0.5 gm orally 3-5 times a day) can be given as an alternative therapy but this is less effective.

Sodium bicarbonate be given in large doses in divided doses.

For treatment of lead encephalopathy 0.1-0.2 g phenobarbitone I/V is useful.

Diet should be low in calcium but high in phosphorus.

LEVORPHANOL (An Opioid)

It is a synthetic opioid used as analgesic.

Clinical Picture and the Management

Same as other with **Methadone** *(Refer page 215)*.

LINDANE (Organochlorine Pesticide)

It is widely used as a pesticide in agriculture, insect control and malarial control programmes. It is moderately toxic among organochlorines with animal oral LD_{50} > 50 mg/kg. Estimated adult lethal dose is 10-30 gm and as little as 1 gm can produce seizures in a child.

Clinical Picture and the Management

Same as with other **Aldrin or DDT** or **Organochlorines** *(Refer page 218)*.

LITHIUM CARBONATE (Anti-depressant and Anti-hypomaniac)

Lithium is commonly indicated for the treatment of bipolar depression.

Lithium is an alkali metal which is distributed throughout the body water and accumulates in cells although distribution from the extracellular to intracellular compartment is relatively slow. **It has a narrow therapeutic index.**

Symptoms of Toxicity

Nausea, vomiting and diarrhoea, ataxia, coarse tremors, drowsiness progressing to coma, mask like face with open eyes, acute renal failure, acute diabetes insipidus, myocardial infarction and polyneuropathy. Hypernatraemia, hypokalemia, ECG shows non-specific ST depression and T wave inversion.

Management

If a large overdose is taken the stomach should be emptied. **To minimize the absorption the sustained release formulations need whole bowel irrigation.**

Frusemide:

Adult: 1 mg/kg at 6 hrs intervals.

Children: 2-3 mg/kg/day PO or 1-2 mg/kg/day IV.

IV fluids:

Adult: 5% dextrose 4-6 liter over 6 hours.

Children: 5% dextrose.

Potassium supplements should be given as required.

Clearance of lithium by peritoneal dialysis is not more than by forced diuresis therefore it is of little value.

Haemodialysis is most efficient method of removing lithium from the intravascular compartment but rebound increase in serum concentrations (upto 100%) can be expected within few hours as the plasma reequilibrates with intracellular fluid. Haemodialysis must therefore be repeated frequently, allowing serum lithium concentration to raise between dialysis.

LIZARD BITES

Indian lizards are non-poisonous. The poison lizards are present only in Mexico and USA.

LORAZEPAM (Benzodiazepine)

It is a sedative hypnotic drug, belonging to benzodiazepine class. It is used in the treatment of anxiety, insomnia, epilepsy and for sedation and amnesia before surgery.

These medicines do not usually cause severe poisoning and unconscious patient normally recovers completely if given medical care.

If these medicines are taken with alcohol it is likely to cause severe poisoning.

Clinical Picture and Management

Same as of other **Benzodiazepines** *(Refer page 73)*.

LUPIN (Plant Toxicity)

L

Lupin lupinus species are widely cultivated decoration plant. Lupin seeds are ingested accidentally by small children that produce toxicity.

Symptoms

Convulsions, respiratory depression, muscular weakness and bradycardia. Anticholinergic symptoms are of shorter duration.

Management

In most cases treatment is not required.

Stomach emptying is indicated if large number of seeds have been ingested.

Gastric Lavage

Activated charcoal: Repeated 70-100 gm activated charcoal is given.

Treatment thereafter is symptomatic.

M

MAGNESIUM HYDROXIDE (Purgative)

It is a purgative given to people who cannot pass stools easily or who pass hard stools.

These tablets look and taste like sweets or chocolate and children may eat them by mistake.

Large amounts of laxatives can cause serious poisoning and death due to dehydration and electrolyte imbalance.

Signs and Symptoms of Toxicity

Diarrhoea, vomiting and abdominal pain, blood in stools.

Fall in blood pressure with rapid pulse.

Unconsciousness.

Management

If the patient is unconscious or drowsy, lay him or her on one side in the recovery position. Check breathing every 10 minutes and keep the patient warm.

If the patient is conscious and alert, give drinks to replace the water lost in the vomit and stools.

It is not necessary to make the patient vomit. If patient is unconscious replace fluids and electrolytes by IV route.

MAGNESIUM HYDROXIDE AND MAGNESIUM SULFATE (Antacid/Purgative)

These are used as antacids and purgatives.

Signs and Symptoms

Large doses can cause diarrhea leading to dehydration.
The absorbed portion can cause serious poisoning and death.
Blood in stools.
Hypotension.
Tachycardia.
Unconsciousness.

Management

If the patient is unconscious or drowsy, lay him or her on one side in the recovery position. Check breathing every 10 minutes and keep the patient warm.

If the patient is conscious and alert, give drinks to replace the water lost in the vomit and stools.

If unconscious administer fluids IV.

MAGNESIUM SULFATE

Used as purgative.

Signs Symptoms and Management

Same as for other **Magnesium hydroxide** *(Refer page 178).*

MALATHION (Organophosphorus compound)

M

It is an active compound present in FINIT, VEGFU MALATOX, AGROMAL, CYTHION, KATHION, MALADAN MALAZENE, LICEL .

It belongs to organophosphorus group of widely used pesticides that may cause acute or chronic poisoning. It is relatively less toxic organophosphorus compound with an LD_{50} of 1000-2800 mg/kg.

Clinical Picture

Same as of other **Organophosphates.** Treat as **Organophosphorus compound toxicity** *(Refer page 219).*

MANGANESE

Manganese intoxication is generally caused by chronic rather than acute exposure. Industrial mining, metal working like smelting and welding are the areas of manganese contamination.

Symptoms

Acute high level manganese inhalation can produce an irritant type of pneumonitis. Chronic toxicity occurs over months or years. The patient usually presents with an psychotic disorders (frequently misdiagnosed as schizophrenia or atypical psychosis). Neurologic toxicity, such as parkinsonism or other extrapyramidal movement disorders, usually appear later.

Management

On ingestion: Inorganic manganese is poorly absorbed from the gastrointestinal tract, therefore lavage is probably not necessary.

On acute inhalation: Remove victim from site of exposure and give supplemental oxygen if available. Treat broncho-spasm and noncardiogenic pulmonary edema, if they occur.

Mild Toxicity

Uneasy feeling, increasing agitation, hallucinations, rest-lessness, moderate writhing of limbs, grinding of teeth, exaggerated limb reflexes, myoclonus.

Chronic intoxication: Psychiatric and neurologic effects are treated with the usual psychiatric and anti-parkinsonian drugs.

M

Management

Maintenance of airway and ventilation is important. If deemed necessary, assisted ventilation with oxygen supplementation may be provided.

Antidotes

EDTA and other chelators have not been proved effective after chronic neurologic damage has occurred. The efficacy of chelators early after acute exposure has not been studied.

MAPROTILINE (Antidepressant)

It is tetracyclic antidepressant. It has the significant advantage over tricyclic antidepressants. **Half life is long 40 hours.**

Symptoms

Mild toxicity: Confusion, blurred vision, flushed dryness of skin and mucosa, sinus tachycardia and hypotension.

Moderate to severe toxicity: Mydrasis, agitation, visual and auditory hallucinations, myoclonus, convulsions, ataxia, coma, hypotension, sinus tachycardia and other brady arrhythmias with prolonged PR and QRS duration (100 m sec). Metabolic acidosis, respiratory insufficiency or arrest, pulmonary edema, oesophageal spasm and urinary retention are other features.

Death occurs due to cardiac arrest and circulatory failure. Death has been reported after ingestion of 2-10 gms but in certain individuals even less than one tenth therapeutic daily dose (75-300 mg) produced severe toxicity.

Management

Induce emesis by mechanical stimulation of the back of the tongue.

Maintain proper airway and ensure adequate oxygenation.

In absence of activated charcoal gastric lavage is indicated.

For controlling seizures administer diazepam.

Or

Lorazepam: 1-2 mg IV over several minutes.

IV fluids to be given according to the needs of the patient.

Sodium bicarbonate: 500-800 ml IV by slow infusion (7.5% v.v.). Aim at maintaining a blood pH of 7.5.

Dobutamine: 2.5-5 ug/kg/min infusion if hypotension is due to loss of cardiac contractility.

Potassium chloride: To be given only if indicated and with monitoring.

Precautions

Do not give antiarrhythmic drugs like quinidine and procainamide as they further decrease AV nodal conduction.

Do not give phenothiazines for treating hyperthermia as their own antichoilinergic action adds to that of the poison.

If possible, avoid high doses of dopamine to treat hypotension as its adrenergic stimulatory effect may increase asthmogenicity and also exacerbate vasodilation.

Treat seizures promptly to prevent hypoxia and lactic acidosis which predispose to developments of ventricular arrhythmias.

Patients should be closely monitored specially for 24 hours after discontinuation of all supportive therapeutic interventions.

Use of phenytoin for seizures control should be avoided as it is likely to increase risk of ventricular tachycardia.

Avoid propranolol and verapamil as they further slow conduction velocity in myocardium, reduce heart rate and lower BP.

Potassium replacement during bicarbonate treatment should be done with caution as hyperkalemia may aggravate antidepressant induced cardiac arrhythmias.

MARIJUANA (Plant Part used for Euphoria)

Marijuana is obtained from the leaves of the plant Cannabis sativa (Indian Hemp) and is usually smoked in cigarettes or pipes. It contains tetrahydrocannabinol. Resin obtained from flowering tops of the plant is called Hashish.

Symptoms

Symptoms appear in 10-20 minutes Subjective effects after smoking a marijuana cigarette include euphoria, palpitations, heightened sensory awareness and altered time perception followed after about 30 minutes by sedation. Relatively severe intoxication results in impaired short term memory, depressonalization visual hallucinations and acute paranoid psychosis.

M

From use of contaminated marijuana infections may occur-Salmonellosis and pulmonary aspergillosis.

Intravenous use of marijuana extract (as cannabis tea) or hash oil may cause dyspnea, abdominal pain, fever, hypotension, shock and disseminated intravascular coagulation. Acute renal failure and cholestatic jaundice are delayed by a few days. CNS symptoms associated with smoking are absent.

Management

Most psychological disturbances may be managed by reassurance possibly along with diazepam or midazolam.

Sinus tachycardia usually does not require treatment but if necessary may be controlled with beta blockers such as propranolol.

Orthostatic hypotension responds to head down position and intravenous fluids.

There is no specific antidote.

On oral ingestion of leaves administer activated charcoal if available. Ipecac induced emesis may be useful for initial treatment at the scene if it can be given within a few minutes of exposure.

Procedures aimed at increasing elimination (such as diuretics haemodialysis) are not effective owing to the large volume of distribution.

Treatment of smokers of marijuana is not necessary.

MECHANICAL IRRITANTS

Powdered glass, glass wool, diamond dust, bunch of pins or thorns or needles, may be ingested for suicidal purposes. These are inert substances but produce symptoms by their mechanical actions on the mucus lining of the gastrointestinal tract.

Symptoms

Abdominal pain and blood in stools.

Management

Bulky food like oat meal, bread, or rice, mashed banana need to be admionstered to enmesh the articles. Followed by laxatives to help their excretion.

Emetics should be avoided.

M

MECLIZINE (Anti histaminic)

It is a H_1 blocker used to treat allergy, travel sickness and cough. It is often available at home therefore children can easily get hold. As a result, its toxicity is common among children.

Signs and Symptoms

Acute intoxication results in symptoms very similiar to those of anticholinergic poisoning.

Clinical Symptoms and Management

Same as for other **Antihistamines** *(Refer page 61).*

MEFENAMIC ACID AND MECLOFENAMATE

Both these drugs inhibit COX and are used as analgesics, antipyretic and anti-inflammatory agents. Symptoms are same as seen with other NSAIDS but diarrhea and abdominal pain are more common. **Mefenamic acid is less effective than aspirin but is more toxic.**

Symptoms

Convulsions (10-20%), muscle twitching, vomiting, and diarrhoea.

Management

Activated charcoal is beneficial.

For treatment of convulsions; give either diazepam or phenytoin in usual doses.

MEPHOSFOLAN (Organophosphate—Insecticide)

Clinical Picture and Management

Same as for other **Organophosphates** *(Refer page 219)*.

MEPROBAMATE (Sedative)

Meprobamate was used as a tranquillizer in 1950s and 1060s. Regular use of meprobamate induces hepatic microsomal enzymes leading to tolerance and consequently acute withdrawal results in obstinence syndrome.

It is no longer available and is currently not used in medicine.

M

MERCURY (Element)

Poisoning due to mercury occurs after ingestion of mercury salts particularly mercuric chloride and accidental or deliberate injection of metallic mercury. Spęcially the commonest accidental exposure to mercury is through ingestion of the bulbs of clinical thermometers by children, but this does not lead to poisoning because of insignificant quantities that are absorbed from the gastrointestinal tract. Toxicity from inhalation of mercury occurs if thermometers break in oven or as occupational hazard in mercury handlers.

Symptoms

After ingestion: Corrosive hemorrhagic gastroenteritis, vomiting, profuse watery diarrhoea, abdominal cramps, limb muscle pain, shock followed by acute renal failure.

After inhalation: Symptoms appear in one hour in the form of cough, chest pain, breathlessness, acute pneumonitis, shivering, generalised weakness, anorexia, joint pains, nausea, increased salivation, headache, irritability, fatigue, memory impairment, sleeplessness, incoordination.

After chronic subcutaneous injections: (Mercurials were used as diuretics) Inflammation, febrile, muscular spasm, stomatitis, abdominal pain, progressive renal failure and death.

Management

Treatment after small quantity of metallic mercury is unnecessary e.g. from thermometer. **Gastric emptying is contraindicated after mercury chloride.**

Management is required if patient has inhaled or taken mercury by parenteral route.

Patient should be shifted immediately if the atmosphere is contaminated with Hg vapour.

Analgesic: May be given according to need.

Surgical excision of subcutaneous mercury should be undertaken to minimize both the local reaction and risk of systemic poisoning.

BAL (Dimercaprol): Chelation therapy to be given promptly when features of systemic poisoning develop regardless of route of exposure. **The drug of choice is dimercaprol for severe inorganic mercury poisoning** in a maximum dose of 5 mg/kg IM followed by 2-5 mg/kg IM every 12-24 hours for 10 days.

Chelation therapy with dimercaprol is advised in symptomatic patients or high level exposures.

For asymptomatic or low level exposure, penicillamine is preferred.

Penicillamine (250 mg PO every 6 hours) may be used alone or following treatment with dimercaprol. The duration of chelation therapy should be determined according to serum and urine concentration of mercury.

It should be used with extreme caution in patients with renal failure.

Hemodialysis should be resorted to in event of renal failure. Chelators may still be used because the dimercaprol mercury complex is still removed by dialysis.

Renal failure to be treated conventionally.

METALDEHYDE (Chemical)

Metaldehyde is used for killing slugs. It is also used as solid fuel. Children and animals are most at risk from accidental poisoning that is rarely serious. Consumption of more than 100 mg/kg body weight may cause serious toxicity. It is uncommon in India

Special risk groups: Pellets are often sold in packs that are easily accessible to children.

If swallowed in large quantities it effects the gut, the brain, the liver and the kidneys.

Symptoms of Toxicity

1-3 hours after ingestion: Nausea, vomiting, abdominal pain, diarrhoea, generalised increase in muscle tone, convulsions, impairment of consciousness and metabolic acidosis.

After two-three days: Jaundice and signs of liver damage, patient passes very little urine showing that kidneys are damaged.

Management

Stomach should be emptied if more than 50 mg/kg is ingested. If swallowed in large quantities make the patient vomit. Give activated charcoal and water to drink.

Patent airway should be maintained.

Convulsions treated with diazepam.

Adult dose—5-10 mg intravenously slowly over a period of 2-3 minutes.

M

Children—0.25-0.4 mg/kg intravenous slowly over a period of 2-3 minutes.

Maintain acid base balance according to individual requirement.

METHADONE (Long Acting Opioid)

It is used to treat withdrawal symptoms of opioids and is given to patients of cancer for relief of pain.

Signs and Symptoms

Signs and symptoms of acute poisoning usually begin within 20-30 min after oral ingestion and are same as other opioids.

Management is also similar to other opioids except that **naloxone needs to be repeated for long time as methadone has long half life and takes longer time to leave body.**

METHANOL (Methyl Alcohol)

Methanol is a common ingredient in many solvents, windshield-washing solutions, duplicating fluids and paint removers. It is sometimes used as an ethanol substitute by alcoholics. Poisoning by methanol is the result of formation of its metabolites—formic and lactic acid—that cause severe acidosis while accumulation of formate results in blindness. Rate of metabolism is independent of methanol concentration in plasma. **A low or nondetectable methanol level does not rule out a serious intoxication in a patient.**

Toxic dose: The fatal oral dose of methanol is estimated to be 30-240 mL (20-150 g). The minimum toxic dose is approximately 100 mg/kg.

Elevated serum methanol levels have been reported even after extensive dermal exposure and concentrated inhalation.

Rate of metabolism is only 1/7th that of ethanol.

Serum methanol levels higher than 20 mg/dL are toxic, and levels higher than 40 mg/dL are very serious.

Symptoms of Toxicity

Symptoms vary according to the time elapsed between ingestion of methanol and hospital presentation.

Latent period of 8-36 hours precedes intoxication.

In the first two hours

Inebriation occurs only if large quantities are ingested.

Acidosis is also not usually present at this stage. However, an osmolar gap of 10 mosm/L is suggestive of methanol poisoning.

After a latent period of 8-36 hours after ingestion:

GIT: Vomiting, severe abdominal pain.

CNS: Headache, vertigo, motor restlessness, seizures and coma.

Ocular: Visual disturbances described as standing in a snowfield and blindness. Fundoscopic examination may reveal optic disc hyperemia, venous enlargement or papilledema.

Skin: Cold clammy extremities.

Respiratory: Dyspnoea, respiration is slow, shallow, gasping and fish mouth. Death usually occurs due to respiratory failure and may be sudden.

Management

The severity of methanol poisoning is proportional to the severity of acidosis and therefore correct acidosis.

Prevent aspiration of fluid, intubate and provide assisted ventilation if deemed necessary.

M

Emesis or gastric lavage is not indicated unless substantial quantity has been ingested and the patient is fully conscious.

a. Ipecac is given within few minutes of presentation (e.g. accidental ingestion by children at home).
b. Gastric lavage is beneficial if performed within 30-35 minutes of ingestion.

Activated charcoal should not be given as it does not absorb methanol and may delay the absorption of orally administered ethanol given as antidote.

Administer glucose:

Adults: 50%, dextrose, 50 ml (25 gm) I.V.

Children: 25% dextrose, 2 ml/kg I.V.

Administer sodium bicarbonate for correction of acidosis.

Dose: 500-800 ml I.V. (7.5 v/v). Maintain blood pH at 7.5 or higher.

Patient should be shifted to a quiet dark room.

Protect eyes from light.

Antidote: Ethanol

Ethanol therapy: It is indicated when:

a. Confirmed history of methanol ingestion.
   Or
b. The osmolar gap > 5 mosm/L and but report on methanol serum levels are not immediately available.
   Or
c. When osmolar gap is greater than 5-10 mosm/L not accounted for by ethanol.

Ethanol can be given orally or intravenously. The intravenous loading dose should be given over a period of 20-30 minutes or longer.

Ethanol Dosing (Adults and Children)

Dose	*Intravenous*		*Oral*	
	5%	10%	50%	95%
Loading	**10** ml/kg	**7-5** ml/kg	**1.5** ml/kg	**0.8-1** mg/kg in 30 min
Maintenance	**2-4** ml/kg/h	**1-2** ml/kg/h	**0.2-0.4** ml/kg/h	**0.32** ml/kg/h
For maintain once during hemodialysis	**4-7** ml/kg/h	**2-3.5** ml/kg/h	**0.4-0.7** ml/kg/h	**0.32** ml/kg/h

If alongwith methanol the patient has also ingested ethanol, then the dose of ethanol needs to be reduced so that the blood ethanol levels do not exceed 100-130 mg/dl. For best results blood ethanol levels be maintained at

100-130 mg/dl. **It is advisable to maintain blood ethanol levels on the higher side (130 mg%) than on lower side (100 mg%) of normal limits.**

Oral doses of ethanol maintenance:

In chronic drinker–0.32 ml/kg/hr.

In non-drinker–0.23 ml/kg/hr.

On an average of 0.27 ml/kg/hr.

Hemodialysis rapidly removes methanol as well as formate and to be continued until serum methanol concentration is less than 20 mg/dl. **It is important to increase ethanol infusion during dialysis.**

Folic acid

Dose: 50 mg IV every 4 hours.

METHIOCARB (A Carbamate Insecticide)

It is used as insecticide. It acts by inhibiting cholinesterase (like organophosphorus compounds but action is short lasting.

Signs, Symptoms and Management

Same as with **Organophosphates** *(Refer page 219)*. **But oximes are not effective and are contraindicated.**

METHOMYL (A Carbamate Insecticide)

Clinical Picture and Management

Same as with **Orgenophosphates** *(Refer page 219)*. **But oximes are not effective and are contraindicated.**

METHOXYCHLOR (Organochlorine Insecticide)

It is widely used as a pesticide in agriculture, insect control and malarial control programs. It is least toxic among organochlorines with animal oral LD_{50} > 1 gm/kg.

Signs, Symptoms and Management

Same as with other **Organochlorines.** Toxicity is therefore treated as per **Organochlorines** *(Refer page 218)*.

METHYL AMPHETAMINE (Amphetamine)

Like amphetamine it too has sympathomimetic activities.

The toxic level of methyl amphetamine is reportedly 1.91 mg/L while for methyl phenidate it is 0.24 mg/L of ritalinic acid which is the principle metabolite.

Clinical Picture and Treatment

Same as that of **Amphetamine** *(Refer page 57).*

METHYL CELLOSOLVE (A Glycol)

It belongs to the group of chemicals called as glycols and are used extensively in industry and other areas. It is also called as ethylene glycol mono methyl ether. Chronic exposure may result in oligospermia.

Signs and Symptoms

Signs and symptoms are like those due to ethylene glycol. Ethanol, folic acid, pyridoxine and thiamine are given as in management of ethylene glycol.

METHYL PHENIDATE (CNS Stimulant Amphetamine Group)

It is central nervous system stimulant with pharmacological profile similar to that of amphetamine with more pronounced effects on mental activities than motor. It is volatile substance of abuse. It is habit forming and there is psychological dependence.

Symptoms of Toxicity

Nervousness, insomnia, dizziness, agitation, psychosis, chorea, palpitations, anginal attacks, arrhythmias, skin rashes, anorexia, visual disturbances, alopecia, anemia, and leucopenia.

Prolonged use in children can suppress growth and exacerbate behavioural disorders.

Management

Stop use.

No specific antidote is available therefore treatment is symptomatic. Activated charcoal is given and in absence of charcoal gastric lavage is done to remove unabsorbed portion of the drug.

Phenothiazines—Specially chlorpromazine and propoxyphene can antagonize its CNS effects.

METHYLENE CHLORIDE (Solvent)

Methylene chloride (dichloro methane) is widely used solvent commonly available in paint. Its prolonged contact with tissue leads to local necrosis but systemic toxicity is usually due to inhalation in less ventilated spaces.

Symptoms of Toxicity

Impairment of consciousness, coma, abdominal pain, joint pains, rashes, altered liver functions, burn lesions in oesophagus.

After prolonged dermal contact: Burns.

On inhalation: Pulmonary oedema.

Management

Gastric emptying is contraindicated.

Treatment is supportive.

Patient should be removed from the contaminated place.

Contaminated clothes should be removed immediately.

Maintain adequate airway.

Acid base balance should be corrected by appropriate methods. Main part of treatment.

Administer oxygen if carboxyhemoglobin concentrations are raised. Hyperbaric oxygen can be used in selected cases but its usefulness is debatable.

Skin lesions should be treated like any other burns.

METOCLOPRAMIDE (Dopaminergic Blocker)

It is selective motility stimulant of gut (prokinetic). It has cholinomimetic activities and is also dopaminergic blocker in CNS. Hastens esophageal clearance rate and raises lower esophageal sphincter pressure along with acceleration of gastric emptying. Large doses are employed in cancer patients for treatment of emesis.

Symptoms

Toxicity is rare but patient may present with uncontrollable chewing movements of mouth and tongue, spasmodic torticollis and oculogyric crises.

Management

Metoclopramide should be stopped.

Diphenhydramine: Administer 2 mg/kg diphenhydramine, maximum dose should not exceed 50 mg/day.

Or

Procyclidine: 5-10 per day mg to be given orally.

Or

Benztropine: 1-2 mg per day either I/M or I/V or orally to be given in case procyclidine is not available.

Route of administration depends on severity.

This stops dystonic reactions in few minutes.

MEVINPHOS (Organophosphate)

It is a highly toxic organophosphorus compound with a LD_{50} of 3-12 mg/kg. Can cause actue as well as chronic toxicity.

Clinical Picture

M

Same as of other organophosphates. Treat as **Organophosphorus poison** *(Refer page 219)*.

MINASERIN (Antidepressant)

Minaserin is a tetracyclic antidepressant that is devoid of anticholinergic properties e.g. dryness of mouth, constipation etc.).

Symptoms of Toxicity

Drowsiness, unconsciousness, CNS depression, hypertension/hypotension, arrhythmias. Patient may not suffer convulsions but epilepsy is worsened.

Management

Activated charcoal (70-100 gms) to be given in repeatedly.

Hemodialysis does not have any value.

Treatment is supportive and symptomatic.

MINOXIDIL (Antihypertensive)

It is an orally effective vasodilator. It dilates arterioles but not veins and is used as antihypertensive agent in patients who do not respond to standard drugs. More often it is used to treat baldness. Serious acute overdoses seldom occur.

Toxic levels: Minimum toxic levels have not been established.

Symptoms of Toxicity

Severe hypotension resulting in dizziness, weakness and syncope, headache, nausea, orthostatic hypotension, warm flushed skin and palpitation, lethargy and ataxia.

Severe hypotension may also result in cerebral and myocardial ischemia and acute renal failure.

Management

If the patient is unconscious or drowsy lay him or her on one side in the recovery position. Check breathing every 10 minutes and keep the patient warm.

Assisted ventilation with oxygen supplementation should be provided if it is necessary.

Vasodilator overdose induced hypotension responds to supine positioning. In case no effect is seen, manage as described below:

a. Fluid therapy must be instituted at the rate of 10-20 ml/kg.
b. Dopamine. Infuse 5 μg/kg/min.

For decontamination, activated charcoal is effective. Gastric emptying is not necessary if activated charcoal is given promptly.

M

MIREX (Organochlorine)

It is widely used as a pesticide in agriculture, insect control and malarial control program. It is moderately toxic among organochlorines with animal oral LD_{50} > 50 mg/kg.

Clinical Picture

Same as with other **Organochlorines** *(Refer page 218)*. Treatment is also on similar lines.

MISTELTOE (Plant Toxin)

There are many plants in this species (Phoradendron and Viscum) that are toxic to man and animals. In Asia Valbum and Var. coloradum are common and are used in traditional systems of medicine.

Symptoms

Vomiting, abdominal pain, diarrhoea, muscle weakness, bradycardia and circulatory failure.

Phorandendron causes hypertension while viscum species produces hypotension.

Fixed and dilated pupils, diplopia and inflammed conjunctiva.

Management

Children who have taken more than 3-5 berries or leaves need to be hospitalized.

Infuse 10-20 mg/kg isotonic fluid but if hypotension persists administer dopamine.

Activated charcoal: Repeated doses of activated charcoal to be given with water.

Calcium gluconate: (Given if there is circulatory failure) - 10-20 ml of calcium gluconate (10%) IV slowly or 5-10 ml of calcium chloride (10%) IV slowly.

Children: 0.2-0.3 ml/kg calcium gluconate (10%) IV slowly or 0.1 to 0.2 ml/kg calcium chloride IV slowly.

Monitor: liver enzymes.

MONOAMINE OXIDASE INHIBITORS (Phenelzine, Isocarboxazid, Tranylcypromine, Nialamide, Proxiazid, Moclobemide)

These drugs are used in treatment of depression not responding to other drugs. Acute toxicity is not common but toxicity due to interactions is serious

Moclobemide differs from other compounds as it causes reversible inhibition of mono amine oxidases and the effect is short lasting. Interactions with food are weak.

In general dose of 4-6 mg/kg or above proves fatal and 2-3 mg/kg is considered potentially life threatening.

Tranylcypromine: Has low therapeutic index, even 170 mg of this drug in an adult resulted in mortality. Therapeutic blood concentrations are 0.1 ml/L while post-mortem blood levels ranged between 0.25-9.0 mg/L.

Phenelzine: 375-1500 mg total dose or 4-6 mg/kg proved fatal.

Nialamide: It is relatively safe and 5 gms and above reported to have resulted in mortality.

Moclobemide: Therapeutic levels range between 0.36 to 3.00 mg/L Toxic levels not known.

Symptoms

Symptoms are due to CNS overactivity.

Even after acute ingestion of the overdose of drugs, it takes 6-24 hours before symptoms are evident. However, if interacting drug/food is taken in the meantime, it may be precipitated immediately.

Severe Toxicity

Severe hypertension that may cause intracranial hemorrhage convulsions, pyrexia, dilated pupils, nystagmus, tachycardia, increased blood pressure, profuse sweating.

Delirium.

Hyperthermia.

Ultimately cardiovascular collapse and multisystem failure cause death.

Serotonin Syndrome

It is characterized by severe rigidity, hyperthermia myoclonic jerking, hyperreflexia and diaphoresis when patients poisoned with MAO inhibitors consume one of the following drugs; **meperidine, dextromethorphan, fluoxetine, paroxetine, sertraline, or tryptophan.**

M

Initial Symptoms

Uneasy feeling, increasing agitation, hallucinations, restlessness, writhing of limbs, grinding of teeth, exaggerated limb reflexes, myoclonus convulsions, pyrexia, dilated pupils, nystagmus, tachycardia, increased blood pressure and profuse sweating.

Management

Treatmemt is mainly supportive and symptomatic.

Ventilatory support may be provided.

Repeated doses of activated charcoal is given for removing unabsorbed portion of the drug.

Dantrolene to be given if there is increase in muscle tone: 1-2 mg/kg IV rapidly may be repeated, as needed every 5-10 min. to a total dose of 10 mg/kg.

Give 1-2 mg/kg IV orally upto maximum of 100 mg 4 times a day for 2-3 days to prevent recurrence of hyperthermia.

Diazepam or phenytoin or phenobarbitone is given to control convulsions.

Hypertension is treated by alpha adrenoreceptor blocking agents such as phentolamine or phenyoxybenzamine.

Haloperidol helps reduce over activity.

Treat hypertension by administering any one of the following drugs:

Phentolamine: 1-5 mg IV (children 0.02-0.1 mg/kg as a bolus) in adults. Repeat at 5-10 minutes intervals (or constant infusion of 0.1-2 mg/min) as needed to lower blood pressure to a desired level (usually <100 mg/Hg diastolic in adults and 80 mm Hg diastolic in children).

Or

Nifedipine: 10 mg sublingually for adults and 0.25-0.5 mg/kg/dose for children.

Do not use extended release formulation for sublingual administration

Or

Nitroprusside Dosage: The average dose is 3 µg/kg/min in children and adults and maximum rate of infusion should not exceed 10 µg/kg/min to avoid risk of acute cyanide toxicity. For preparation of the intravenous solution, dissolve 50 mg of sodium nitroprusside in 3 ml of 5% dextrose and dilute this solution in 5% dextrose to achieve a concentration of 200, 100 or 50 µg/ml, respectively. Initiate treatment with 0.3 µg/kg/min and titrate the dose to a desired effect.

M

Nitroprusside solution is photosensitive and therefore, the bottle and intravenous tubing should be protected from light.

It should only be used in emergency or intensive care setting. Blood pressure should be monitored continuously or frequently.

In case, tachycardia is also present, add one of the following to the above mentioned drugs.

Propranolol: 0.02-0.1 mg/kg IV

Esmolol: 25-100 µ/kg/min IV

Labetolol: 0.2-0.3 mg/kg IV

Do not use beta blockers alone for treatment of hypertension as it might result in paradoxical rise in BP.

In case of abnormal neurological findings, a CT scan is advisable to rule out stroke and neurologist should be consulted.

Convulsions Should be managed as described below:

Diazepam: should be given in undiluted form and closely monitor blood pressure and respiration.

Followed by:

Phenytoin.

Or

Phenobarbitone.

In case of repeated convulsions curarization is indicated

Treat hyperthermia by external cooling, as this is the most efficient way of cooling. Iced gastric and colonic lavage or even ice-water immersion can also be carried out. In case shivering occurs as a consequence of cooling, use diazepam (0.1-0.2 mg/kg IV) or midazolam (0.05-0.1 mg/kg IV).

For treating serotonin syndrome, Combination external cooling and diazepam take care of this syndrome.

Monitor temperature, vital signs and ECG for a minimum of 6 hours as poisoning manifests late in asymptomatic patients and admit all symptomatic patients for continous monitoring for at least 24 hours.

Dantrolene is given if muscle tone is extreme.

MONSTERA (Plant)

This is decorative house plant. Poisoning with this plant is most common in children.

Symptoms on Ingestion

Burning pain in lips and mouth, hypersalivation inflammation of buccal mucosa, lips, tongue and swollen palate with difficulty in swallowing. Respiratory obstruction, retrosternal pain and oesophageal necrosis are other features of poisoning.

Management

Treatment is symptomatic.

Advise patient to suck ice and drink milk.

Antacid: 5-10 ml four hourly.

Ranitidine

Adult: 50 mg IV 6-8 hourly. Children: 1.25-2 mg/kg/d. Maximum dose should not exceed 300 mg/day.

Endotracheal intubation (if possible) or tracheostomy is done if there is serious respiratory obstruction.

Corticosteroids: May be given but their value in reducing the oedema has not been assessed.

MORPHINE (Opium Alkaloid)

It is a natural alkaloid of opium (unripe)—Paper umsomniferum. It is used as analgesic in patients not responding to NSAIDs and in terminally ill patients. Use of this highly effective analgesic is restricted because of high addiction liability.

Codeine as well as heroin too are converted to morphine in the body. Tolerance develops to euphoric effect and the addicts continue to increase the dose leading to fatal outcome. Poisoning is often encountered in addicts, and in suicidal cases both in rural areas (opium intake) and urban areas (injectable morphine). It is popular drug for sucide among paramedical and medical staff.

However, because of its euphoric activity its misuse is prevalent and toxicity is often reported.

Sign and Symptoms of acute poisoning usually begin within 20-30 min after oral ingestion and within minutes following parenteral administration.

Symptoms of Toxicity

Shallow breathing with depressed respiratory rate, coma, pinpoint pupils, bradycardia, hypotension, hypothermia, decreased urinary output and gastrointestinal motility. Respiratory depression may lead to hypoxia, cyanosis, convulsions, bronchospasm, pulmonary edema and respiratory arrest. Deaths in opiod poisoning are due to respiratory depression and cardiorespiratory arrest.

Poisoning due to morphine is clinically diagnosed by the presence of **pinpoint pupils, associated with respiratory depression, hypothermia and hypotension.**

Management

Chemical laboratory analysis of urine, blood and a gastric output for presence of opioid is useful diagnostic tool.

Maintain proper ventilation and put the patient on artificial respiration, if needed.

IV fluids are given according to need. Morphine has emetic effect and therefore dehydration is a possibility.

Dopamine: 4-6 ug/kg/min IV is given to treat hypotension.

Gastric lavage is done to remove morphine.

Activated charcoal: Slurry aqueous or mixed with sorbitol is helpful even though morphine is given parenterally.

Specific Antidote

Naloxone

Adult and children dose: 0.4 to 2.0 mg IV. Repeat as needed to reverse signs and symptoms of toxicity.

Neonates: Initial dose is 10-30 μg/kg IV. If no response is observed after 10 mg of naloxone have been administered diagnosis of opioid induced poisoning should be questioned.

Diazepam is given only if patient has convulsions.

MOUSE BITES (Animal Toxicity)

Most mice are not venomous but act as carriers of infection. Shrews (small mouse like creature that looks like a mouse) are often seen in residential areas in India and are venomons yet bites due to shrews have not been reported to cause toxicity.

MUSHROOMS (Food Poisoning)

M

Amanita phalloides (the death cap mushroom) is the most common cause (almost 90%) of deaths associated with mushroom poisoning.

When taking the history from the patient with suspected mushroom poisoning following features need to be considered:

a. The interval between ingestion and onset of symptoms.
b. The number and type of mushroom eaten (it is important because edible and poisonous type often grow closely).
c. If alcohol was taken at the time of eating the mushrooms.
d Onset of symptoms and their sequence.
e. Whether or not the mushrooms cooked before eating, because some toxins (e.g. haemolysins and gastrointestinal irritants) are inactivated by heat while others (specially those with more serious effects) are thermostable.

Symptoms with most common eaten mushrooms (Entoloma sinuatum, Boletus santanas, Russula species, Nalonea sericea, Poxillus involutes, Agarices xanthedermus): produce nausea, vomiting, diarrhoea soon after ingestion.

Diagnosis regarding type of mushroom can be made from time of onset of symptoms.

After over 2 hours of ingestion (Clitocybe, Inocybe, Psilocybe, Panacolus sp and Amantia muscaria and Amanita pantherima): Profuse sweating, salivation, vomiting, abdominal colic, diarrhoea, rhinorrhoea, blurred vision, hallucinations without impairment of consciousness.

After 12 hours of ingestion (Amanita phalloides, A. verna, A. virosa and some species of Galerina): Severe vomiting, abdominal cramps, profuse watery diarrhoea. **0.1 mg/kg of Amanita phaloides causes death.**

Upto 24 hours (Coprinus atramentarius): Flushing, sweating, nausea immediately after alcohol consumption.

72 hours or more (Cortinarius species): Thirst polyuria leading to renal failure.

Management

If breathing stops, give mouth to mouth respiration, and cardiac massage if the heart stops.

If the patient is unconscious or drowsy lay him or her in a quiet dimly lit place, protected from light.

M

If patient had vomiting nausea, diarrhoea then he/she to be treated with available antiemetic and anti diarrhoeal.

Intravenous fluids to be administered for correction of electrocyte imbalance.

If patient had symptoms after 2 hours of ingestion and cholinergic effects are present atropine should be given.

Adult dose: 2-5 mg IV give slowly and repeated till signs of atropinisation appear.

For other varieties of mushrooms. Treat patient symptomatically.

N

NALTREXONE (Opioid Antagonist)

It is similar to naloxone but is more potent. It is used for treating addicts as is suppresses symptoms of morphine administration.

It differs from nalaxone as it is orally effective. In addition it suppresses alcohol urge.

Symptoms

Normal doses do not produce any subjective feelings.

High doses cause unpleasant feelings in some individuals which pass off and do not require treatment.

NAPHTHALENE

Naphthalene balls are used to protect clothing from insects and toxicity results from accidental ingestion by children and intentional by adults.

Signs and Symptoms

If swallowed:

Nausea, vomiting, diarrhoea and abdominal pain.

Sweating.

Fever.

Jaundiced skin.

Urine becomes dark and may contain blood. Anuria may develop.

Convulsions may occur followed by unconsciousness.

In patients with G6PD deficiency naphthalene ingestion is likely to cause hemolysis.

Treatment

Add 100 meq of sodium bicarbonate to each litre of 5% dextrose and infuse.

NAPTHA (Petroleum Distillate)

It is one of the petroleum distillates. Though chemically different toxicity produced is similar in symptoms to petrol products.

Symptoms

Vomiting is common but not necessary. Diarrhoea is uncommon.

There may be excitement, but in severe poisoning drowsiness is seen which may lead to coma.

The most common complication of this poisoning is pulmonary pathology which occurs in almost 60% of the cases and results from aspiration of the poison into the bronchial tree. This results into cough, choking, wheezing and breathlessness.

Clinical evidence of respiratory involvement is usually evident within few minutes after poisoning but in some cases it may be delayed for hours but not more than a day. Severe poisoning can cause hemorrhagic pulmonary oedema which is fatal within 24 hours. Pneumonitis in most of the cases involves two or more lobes and is peripheral in distribution. Fever and polymorph leukocytosis are common.

Rare complications include pneumatocele formation, intravascular hemolysis and renal failure.

Diagnosis of hydrocarbon ingestion may be confirmed by finding a double gastric level on the X-ray of the abdomen taken in the erect position.

Management

Gastric emptying is useful if sufficiently large amount of the poison has been ingested provided patient is sufficiently alert so that he can cough effectively and second the airway should be protected by inserting a cuffed entotracheal tube.

Indications for Gastric Emptying

a. If the amount of ingested poison is more than 1ml/kg of body weight.

   Or

b. If there is suspicion that solution ingested contained another toxin (such as pesticide) in addition.

   Or

c. Signs of serious poisoning are evident.

Antibiotics should be given in only those patients who develop secondary bacterial infections.

If cyanosis is present, oxygen may be necessary. Intermittant positive pressure is indicated for patients with pulmonary oedema.

NIALAMIDE (Antidepressant-MAO Inhibitor)

It is used as an antidepressant and serious toxicity results from overdose or due to interactions with certain other drugs or foods.

Toxic dose

Ingestion of even 2-3 mg/kg of the drug may be life threatening. **Because of irreversible inhibition of the enzyme, adverse drug interactions may occur for upto 2 weeks after discontinuing them.**

Signs and Symptoms

Even after acute ingestion of the overdose of nialamide, it takes 6-24 hours before symptoms are evident. However, if interacting drug/food is taken in the meantime, it may be precipitated immediately.

Mild Toxicity

Anxiety, headache and tremors.
Flushing and sweating.
Myoclonus and hyperreflexia.
Shivering, tachypnea.
Moderate degree hypertension or orthostatic hypotension.
Weight gain.

Severe Toxicity

Severe hypertension.
Intracranial hemorrhage due to hypertension.
Delirium.
Hyperthermia.
Cardiovascular collapse and multisystem failure are the causes of death.

Serotonin Syndrome

It is characterized by severe rigidity, hyperthermia myoclonic jerking, hyperreflexia and diaphoresis when patient poisoned with nialamide consumes one of the following: **meperidine, dextromethorphan, fluoxetine, paroxetine, sertraline, or tryptophan.**

N

Severe hyperpyrexia, restlessness, coma and hypotension occur if given with pethidine.

Management

Maintenance of airway and ventilation is important. If deemed necessary, assisted ventilation with oxygen supplementation may be provided.

Treat hypertension by the use of any one of the following drugs:

Phentolamine: 1-5 mg IV (children 0.02-0.1 mg/kg) as a bolus. Repeat at 5-10 minutes intervals (or constant infusion of 0.1-2 mg/min) as needed to lower blood pressure to a desired level (usually <100 mg/Hg diastolic in adults and 80 mm Hg diastolic in children). **Or**

Nifedipine: 10 mg sublingually for adults and 0.25-0.5 mg/kg/dose for children. Do not use extended release formulation for sublingual administration. **Or**

Nitroprusside: It should only be used in emergency or intensive care setting. Blood pressure should be monitored frequently.

N

Dosage: The average dose is 3 µg/kg/min in children and adults and maximum rate should not exceed 10 µg/kg/min to avoid risk of acute cyanide toxicity. For preparation of the intravenous solution, dissolve 50 mg of sodium nitroprusside in 3 ml of 5% dextrose and dilute this solution in 5% dextrose to achieve a concentration of 200, 100 or 50 µg/ml respectively. Initiate with 0.3 µg/kg/min and titrate the dose to a desired effect. **In case no effect on blood pressure is seen, use an alternative drug.**

Nitroprusside solution is photosensitive and, therefore, the bottle and intravenous tubing should be protected from light.

In case, tachycardia is also present, add one of the following to the above mentioned treatment:

Propranolol: 0.02-0.1 mg/kg IV or

Esmolol: 25-100 µ/kg/min IV or

Labetolol: 0.2-0.3 mg/kg IV.

Do not use beta blockers alone for treatment of hypertension as it might result in paradoxical rise in BP.

In case of abnormal neurological findings, a CT scan is advisable to rule out stroke and neurologist should be consulted.

Convulsions should be managed by **diazepam** given in undiluted form with close monitoring of blood pressure and respiration.

Followed by either **Phenytoin or Phenobarbitone.**
Treat hyperthermia by external cooling.

For treating serotonin syndrome, use diazepam for controlling seizures as described above and apply external cooling.

Continously monitor temperature and vital signs of ECG for a minimum of 6 hours in asymptomatic and admit all symptomatic patients for continuous monitoring.

NICOTINE (Active Principal of Tobacco)

Nicotine is ingested in the form of tobacco and nicotine chewing gum. Nicotine poisoning is not uncommon amongest children. Most individuals who consume 3 cigarettes at a stretch, at the end of each smoking event will have toxic symptoms.

Symptoms

Vomiting and nausea are the most common symptoms and may be accompanied with agitation, hyperactivity, tachycardia, abdominal pain, drowsiness, muscle weakness and jerking of the limbs (less common).

N

Rarely convulsions, respiratory depression and dysarrhythmias may occur. Pupils may be wide or very small.

Management

Perform gastric lavage (if 5 whole cigarettes or 8 stubs or 5 pieces of gum have been ingested).

Adult: 150-200 ml of lukewarm water/saline.

Children: 50-100 ml of lukewarm water/saline.

Give activated charcoal:

Further treatment is symptomatic.

NITRATES AND NITRITES (Antianginal)

Organic nitrates are widely used as vasodilators for the treatment of ischemic heart disease and heart failure. In addition, **bismuth subnitrate, ammonium nitrate and silver nitrate** are used as anti-diarrhoeal, diuretic and for topical use in burn respectively. **Sodium nitrite and nitrates** are used in preserving canned foods and may be present in high concentrations in some well waters.

Symptoms of Toxicity

Headache, skin flushing and orthostatic hypotension with reflex tachycardia are the most common adverse effects of nitrates and nitrites that occur commonly.

Workers or patients regularly exposed to nitrates may develop tolerance and may suffer angina or myocardial infarction owing to rebound coronary vasoconstriction upon sudden withdrawal of the drug.

Management

Maintain airway and assist ventilation if necessary. Administer supplemental oxygen.

On ingestion: Administer activated charcoal if available. Ipecac induced emesis may be useful for initial treatment at the scene. Gastric emptying is not necessary for small ingestion if activated charcoal can be given promptly.

Nitrate overdose induced hypotension usually responds to supine positioning. In case no effect is seen, start fluid therapy with Dopamine. Infuse 4-10 μg/kg/min.

Symptomatic methemoglobinemia may be treated with **methylene blue.** It is indicated if patient has symptoms or signs of hypoxemia (e.g. dyspnoea, confusion, chest pain) or methemoglobinemia > 30%.

N

Dosage (adults and children): 1-2 mg/kg (0.1-0.2 ml/kg of 1% solution) IV slowly over 5 minutes. May be repeated in 30-60 minutes. If no response occurs, do not repeat dosing.

In case of toxicity due to inhalation, remove the victim from the site of exposure and administer supplemental oxygen.

Skin and eyes: Remove contaminated clothing and wash with copious water. Irrigate exposed eyes with water or saline.

Hemodialysis and hemoperfusion are not effective. Severe methemoglobinemia in infants not responsive to methylene blue therapy may require exchange transfusion.

NITRIC ACID (Strong Acid-Corrosive)

Esophageal mucosa is relatively resistant but gastric mucosa is sensitive. Nitric acid is less corrosive than sulphuric acid. It coagulates proteins. Fumes of nitric acid cause irritation of eyes, dyspnea etc and may cause death immediately due to suffocation or later from pulmonary oedema or pneumonia.

It stains skin yellow which is due to formation of xanthoprotric acid.

Fatal dose 10-15 ml.

Fatal period 12-24 hours.

Symptoms of Toxicity

In case of ingestion: Severe burning pain in the mouth, throat, abdomen, dysphagia, gastritis, vomiting, diarrhoea (bloody, mucoid) hypotension with cold clammy skin and rapid pulse. Metabolic acidosis, hemolysis, massive fluid and electrolyte shifts result in hyperkalemia, hyperphosphatemia, hypocalcemia and hyperchloremia.

In case of inhalation: Cough, dyspnea, pleuritic chest pain, pulmonary oedema, frothy sputum, hemoptysis, bronchospasm, pain in eyes, swelling and lacrimation.

In case of eye exposure: Irritation, pain, lacrimation, swelling, chemosis, photophobia, corneal erosin and perforation, Necrosis of conjunctiva and cornea may ultimately occur.

In case of dermal exposure: Thickness of skin with burning pain, irritation, redness, blistering and ulceration.

Management

In case of inhalation: Patient should be shifted to fresh air.

In case of eye exposure: Irrigate with large volumes of 0.9% normal saline or water for 15 minutes or more depending upon severity.

Wash affected skin with copious amounts of water or mild soap solution.

In case of Ingestion:

Do not induce vomiting. Do not give gastric lavage.

Administer water or milk with a view to dilute acid.

Administer IV fluids—Amount to be determined depending upon the degree of hydration. Vasopressors can be added if required

Antibiotics to be given if there is suspicion of infection or in presence of perforation.

Perform endoscopy within first 24 hours.

Perform chest X-ray for detecting mediastinitis or GI perforation.

Perform laparotomy in case endoscopy reveals grade B burns or necrosis of oesophagus or stomach or if signs and symptoms of GI perforation are present at the time of admission.

Do not give excessive amount of milk or water as these provoke vomiting.

Do not give carbonated beverages or bicarbonate for neutralization.

NITROGEN OXIDES

Nitrogen oxides are dangerous chemical gases commonly released from nitrous or nitric acid from reaction between nitric acid and organic materials and from burning of nitrocellulose and many other products. Exposure to nitrogen oxides occur in performing certain techniques such as electric arc welding, electroplating and engraving.

Symptoms

Nitrogen oxides are poorly water soluble therefore, there is very little upper respiratory irritation at low levels. With more concentrated exposures, upper respiratory symptoms such as burning eyes, sore throat and painful brassy cough may occur.

Management

N

Observe patient closley for signs of upper airway obstruction and intubate the trachea and assist ventilation if necessary. Administer humified oxygen.

Observe symptomatic victims for a minimum of 24 hours after exposure and treat chemical pneumonia and non-cardiogenic pulmonary edema if they occur.

Administration of corticosteroids has been recommended, but without convincing evidence.

Treat methemoglobinemia with methylene blue.

Rescured should wear breathing apparatus and wear chemical protective clothing and workers involved int he indutry involving nitrons oxide to must wear maski.

On inhalation: Remove victim from exposure immediately and give supplemental oxygen.

Exposure of Skin and Eyes: Remove any wet clothing and flush exposed eyes with copious water or saline.

NITROPRUSSIDE (Vasodilator)

It is a short acting parenterally administered vasodilator used to treat severe hypertension and cardiac failure. It is also used to induce hypotension for certain surgical procedures. Toxicity may occur with acute high dose nitroprusside treatment or with prolonged infusions.

Symptoms

The most common effect is hypotension, which is often accompanied by reflex tachycardia.

Poisoning is accompanied by headache, hyperventilation, anxiety, agitation, seizures and metabolic acidosis.

It may also cause somnolence, confusion, delirium, tremors and hyperreflexia. Seizures and coma may rarely occur with severe toxicity.

Methemoglobinemia occurs rarely and is usually mild.

Management

Maintain patent airway and assist ventilation if necessary. Administer supplemental oxygen.

For treatment of hypotension, stop the infusion immediately and administer intravenous fluids or even pressors, if necessary. Raise foot end of the bed.

Administer Sodium thiosulfate

Hemodialysis may accelerate thiocyanate elimination and is especially useful in patients with renal failure.

NITRAZEPAM (Benzodiazepine)

Used as sedative and hypnotic.

Symptoms

Mild drowsiness, ataxia, weakness.

Moderate to severe: Apathy, dizziness, lethargy, slurred speech, partial ptosis, nystagmus, response to verbal stimuli may be intact. Hypotension and respiratory depression.

Management

Specific: Flumazenil

Adult—0.2 mg over 30 sec. IV. Repeat at 20 minutes intervals. Maximum dose should not exceed 3 mg in an hour except in profound coma. Flumazenil has short half life therefore needs to be repeated. **Administration of flumazenil can produce convulsion, bradycardia, ventricular arrhythmias and complete heart block.** To reduce adverse reactions of this antidote it is desirable that it be given by an experienced person and hypoxia, hypotension and arrhythmias should be corrected before giving this drug. **Its use should be avoided in patients with history of convulsions or who have consumed tricyclic antidepressants.**

Benzodiazepines are not dialysable.

Perform gastric lavage.

Administer activated charcoal and repeat without purgative every four hours.

For treating convulsions:

Give Phenytoin or Phenobarbitone:

Ensure adequate oxygenation, provide ventilatory support if required.

IV fluids—volume to be determined by the condition of the patient.

Dopamine to be given (4-10 μg/kg/min) intravenously for correction of hypotensive.

NON STEROIDAL ANTI INFLAMMATORY DRUGS (NSAIDs) (Salicylates, Phenacetin, Paracetamol, Phenylbutazone, Indomethacin, Sulindac, Declofenac, Ketorolac, Ibuprofen, Fenoprofen, Naproxen, Ketoprofen, Perofen, Flufenamic acid, Mefenamic acid, Piroxicam, Nimsulide, and Nambutone)

N

Drugs and Their Trade Names

Drugs	*Trade names*
Salicylic acid	Derobin, Dipsalic, Mycodern, Pragmatar
Methyl salicylate	Ethnorub, Flamar cream, Kilpane-oil, Systa flam cream
Acetylsalicylic acid	Aspirin, Cardiwell plus, Dapresal P, Disprin, E-prin, Myoral, Tapal, Thrombosprin, Tuxyne etc.
Diclofinac	Bren, Brufen, Combiflam, Duoflam, Einflam, Febrafen, Fenlong, Ferpar, Flexon, Ibuclin, Ibudoss, Ibuflamar, Ibugesic, Ibugin, Ibusynth, Inflapen, Norswel, Novalgin, Rofiflam, Synol, Tribusynth and Zypar
Ketoprofen	Maxigesic plus, Ostofen, Profemid
Mefenamic acid	Dysmen, Meftal, Ponstan, Kapseals
Naproxen	Artagen, Nalyxan, Naprosy
Oxyphenbuta-zone	Buta-proxyron, Butadex, Flamar P, Oxalgin, Systaflam, Tromalgin

Contd...

Contd...

Drugs	*Trade names*
Phenylbuta-zone	Butapred
Piroxicam	Brexic, Dolonex, Inflavan, Minicam, Ostoden, Piricam, Pirox, Puxicam.

NSAIDs are widely used for their analgesic and anti-inflammatory properties. They are found in a variety of prescriptions and over the counter analgesics, cold preparations and topical keratolytic products (Salicylates).

Symptoms

Patients may become intoxicated following acute accidental or suicidal overdose or as a result of chronic repeated overmedication for several days.

A. **Acute ingestion:** Vomiting occurs shortly after ingestion followed by hyperpnea, tinnitus and lethargy. Mixed respiratory alkalemia and metabolic acidosis are apparent when arterial blood gases are determined. With severe toxicity—coma, seizures and hypoglycemia may occur. Death is due to central nervous system failure and cardiovascular collapse.

Mefanamic acid over dose is associated with serious convulsions—a feature that is seen in 10-20% of patients. Muscle twitching of short duration may also be present. Unlike salicylate, poisoning due to fanamic acid is associated with diarrhoea. Hyponatremia has been reported in new born after maternal poisoning. However the drug has short half life.

Ibuprofen, on the other hand, is relatively safe and ingestion of 100 mg/kg is not likely to produce symptoms. Clinical picture resembles that of salicylates but liver and renal functions may get affected. Arylpropionic acid derivatives such as **ibuprofen, naproxen, Ketoprofen, fenoprofen, flubiprofen and oxaprozin** are better tolerated. Indole and Indene acetic derivatives such as **indomethacin, sulindac and etodolac** are relatively more toxic as compared to arylpropionic acid derivatives.

Indomethacin is highly toxic and 20% of the patients discontinue treatment because of toxicity. In addition to toxicity seen with salicylates it also produces pancreatitis and frontal headache.

Para-aminophenol derivatives such as acetaminophen and phenacetin are likely to cause hepatotoxicity

N

B. **Chronic intoxication:** Victims are usually young children or the elderly suffer confusion, dehydration and metabolic acidosis.

Gastric ulceration is common.

Management

Maintain the airway and assist ventilation if necessary. Administer supplemental oxygen.

Treat coma, seizures, pulmonary edema and hyperthermia if they occur.

Treat metabolic acidosis with intravenous sodium bicarbonate.

Replace fluid and electrolyte deficits caused by vomiting and hyperventilation with intravenous crystalloid solutions. Should be cautious with fluid therapy, because excessive fluid administration may contribute to pulmonary edema.

There is no specific antidote for any NSAID except paracetamol.

N

Decontamination is not necessary for patients with chronic intoxication.

Ipecac induced emesis may be useful for initial treatment of acute toxicity if it can be given within 30 minutes of exposure. Gastric lavage is not necessary after small ingestions.

However in acute poisoning administer **activated charcoal** and a cathartic orally or by gastric tube.

Urinary alkalization, hemodialysis, hemoperfusion and repeat dose activated charcoal therapy are effective means of removal of salicylates.

Treat hypotension by dopamine. Vitamin K_1 is given for patients with bleeding.

Adult: K_1 10-25 mg/day.

Children: 5-10 mg/day further dose to be adjusted according to prothrombin time.

NORTRIPTYLINE (TCA—Antidepressant)

Symptoms

Mild: Confusion, blurred vision, flushed dry skin and mucosa, sinus tachycardia, hypotension.

Moderate to severe: Mydrasis, agitation, visual and auditory hallucinations, myoclonus convulsions, ataxia, coma, hypotension, sinus tachycardia or brady arrhythmias with prolonged PR and QRS duration (100 m sec) metabolic acidosis, respiratory insufficiency or arrest, pulmonary edema, oesophageal spasm and urinary retention.

Deaths in tricyclic antidepressants are due to cardiac arrest and circulatory failure.

Management

Laboratory tests advised are:

ECG monitoring.

Blood gases, bicarbonate and serum pH.

Serum electrolytes.

Quantitative test for TCA.

Induce emesis by mechanical stimulation at the back of the tongue.

Place a spoon in patient's mouth in case of seizures to prevent injury to tongue.

Ensure adequate oxygenation.

Maintain proper airway.

Nasopharangeal suction to be done.

Gastric lavage:

Adult: 150-200 ml of lukewarm water or normal saline per wash.

Child: 50 to 100 ml of normal saline in children below 5 years may be repeated and repeat without purgative every 4-6 hours in a dose of 0.5 gm/kg every 6 hours.

Activated Charcoal

Child: 15-30 gm orally mixed with water (single dose) and repeat 0.25 gm/kg every 4-6 hours.

Diazepam is given to control convulsions.

Diazepam should be given in undiluted form and closely monitor blood pressure and respiration. **Or**

Lorazepam: 1-2 mg IV given slowly over several minutes.

Followed by:

Phenytoin

Or

Phenobarbitone

Administer IV fluids according to the need of the patient.

Adult: 100 ml of 50% dextrose.

Child: 0.5-1 gm/kg of 25% dextrose.

Sodium bicarbonate: 500-800 ml IV slow infusion (7.5% v.v), to maintain a blood pH of 7.5.

Dobutamine: 2.5-1.5 ug/kg/min infusion to if hypotension is due to loss of inotropy.

Potassium chloride: (If indicated) with monitoring.

For precautions refer **Antidepressants.**

O

OLEANDER PLANT (White Nerium oderum)

This plant contains poisons that affect heart and if taken in large quantities can cause death. It is cerebrocardiac poison. All parts of plant are toxic. Roots/seeds of this plant are used as abortifacient in some areas. For abortfacient effect it is either ingested or applied locally on the cervix of the uterus.

It is used for suicidal purposes in India.

Toxicity is due to presence of three glycosides—Neriodrin, Neriodorein and Karabin. Fatal dose is 250 gm of plant or approximately 16.6 gms of the root.

Fatal period is 24-36 hours.

Special Risk Groups

The bright flowers are attractive to children and can be cause of accidental-poisoning.

Symptoms ot Toxicity

Burning sensation of oral cavity, tingling of tongue, dryness of throat, nausea, vomiting, diarrhoea, giddiness, dizziness, confusion, delirium, hypertension in early stage is followed by hypotension, pale and cold extremities, bradycardia and AV block, ST segment depression, atrial and ventricular fibrillation and ventricular tachycardia.

After Inhalation: Acute haemolysis occurs after prolonged inhalation. Cardiotoxicity occurs after inhalation of smoke from burning of plant.

Dermal: Irritation and inflammation of the skin.

Management

Laboratory tests advisable: ECG and serum K^+ levels.

There is **no specific antidote**

Cholestyramine/colestipol given orally to reduce absorption of toxin in the gut.

Supportive: Manage airway and provide artificial oxygen and maintain circulation.

Perform gastric lavage with lukewarm water or saline.

Activated charcoal can be given.

Sorbitol:

Adult: 1-5 gm/kg orally as 70% solution upto a maximum 150 gm.

Children: 1-1.5 gm/kg/dose as a 35% solution orally upto a maximum of 50 gm dose.

Potassium chloride to be given if serum K^+ is low:

Adult: 0.5-1.0 mEq/min in 0.9% or 0.45% saline.

Children: 0.3 mEq/kg/dose/hr.

Administer sodium bicarbonate:

Adult: 2.5 mEq/kg over 4-8 hours depending on acidosis.

Children: Initial dose; 1 mEq/kg after that half give the total dose every 10 minutes till correction of pH.

Atropine:

Adult: 0.6 mg IV maximum dose 2 mg/day with continuous ECG monitoring.

Lidocaine:

Adult: Bolus: 0.7-1.4 mg/kg.

Infusion: 14-57 ug/kg/min with continuous ECG monitoring.

Child: Bolus: 1 mg/kg.

Infusion: 30 ug/kg/min with continuous ECG monitoring.

Or

Phenytoin:

Adult: 100 mg/dose IV slowly every 5 minutes upto 1 gm or until arrhythmias are controlled or nystagmus develops along with constant cardiac monitoring.

Child: 5 mg/kg/dose given at the rate of 40 mg/min with ECG monitoring.

OMETHOATE (Organophosphate—Insecticide)

It is organophosphate compound used as insecticide.

Symptoms and Management

Same as with other **Organophosphates** *(Refer page 219)*.

OPIOIDS/OPIUM (Plant)

Opioids (In alphabetical order)

Buprenorphine

Codeine

O

Dextromormide
Dextropropoxyphene
Dihydrocodeine
Diphenoxylate
Dipopanone
Etorphine
Heroin (Diacetylmorphine)
Hydromorphine
Methadone
Morphine
Nalbuphine
Opium
Oxymorphone
Pentazocine
Phenazocine
Pethidine

Brand names of officially avoidable opioids.

Opioid	*Brand name*
Codeine	Bronolax, Ephedrex, Exiplon, MIT's linetus, Codeinae Co, Phensedyl, Zimalgin.
Dextropropoxyphene	Bren Px, Butaproxyvon Corbutyl, Daprisal P, Dexovon, Ibudess, Proxyvon, Spasmoproxyvon, Walgesic, Wygesic.
Diphenoxylate	Lomofen, Lomotil.
Loperamide	Imodium, Imosec S, Imozol, Jetosec S, Nilamide, Ridol.
Noscapine pentazocine	Tusq, Tuxyne, Dymic, Foracet, Fortagesic, Fortioin, Pentawin, Sosegon.
Methadone	
Pethidine	
Fentanyl	

Symptoms of Toxicity

Signs and symptoms of acute poisoning usually begin within 20-30 min after oral ingestion.

Shallow breathing with depressed respiratory rate, coma, pin point pupils, bradycardia, cardiac arrhythmias, hypotension, hypothermia, convulsions, decreased urinary output and gastrointestinal motility. Respiratory depression may lead to hypoxia, cyanosis, bronchospasm, pulmonary edema and respiratory arrest. Deaths in opiod poisoning are due to respiratory depression and cardiorespiratory arrest.

Cardiac contractile activity is reduced by propoxyphene metabolites.

Speed of onset of clinical features depends on dose and route of administration, but dextro-propoxyphene on oral administration produces quick effects (severe coma, convulsions and respiratory depression).

Management

Chemical laboratory analysis of urine, blood and a gastric output shows presence of alkaloid.

Clinical picture of a drunk patient closely resembles that of an opioid. However in case of opioid poisoning pupils are constructed. Maintain proper ventilation.

Put the patient on artificial respiration if needed.

IV fluids.

Dopamine: 2-10 ug/kg/min IV.

Gastric lavage.

Activated charcoal: Slurry, aqueous or mixed with sorbitol.

Adult: 30 to 100 gms.

Children: 10 to 30 gms.

Infant: 1-2 g/kg.

Specific antidote:

Intravenous infusion of naloxone is recommended for treatment of methadone toxicity.

Naloxone: Dose for adult and children dose 0.4 to 2.0 mg IV repeated if needed to reverse signs and symptoms of toxicity.

Neonates: Initial dose 10-30 ug/kg IV.

If no response is observed after 10 mg of naloxone has been administered—diagnosis of opioid induced poisoning should be questioned.

Infusion is indicated in poisoning with long acting opioids. Continuous IV infusion of 2/3 of initial bolus dose of naloxone on hourly basis. Monitor respiratory rate. CVP carefully during infusion.

Diazepam (To be administered in case of convulsions):

In adults: 5-10 mg IV initially at a maximum rate of 5 mg/min.

ORAL CONTRACEPTIVES

These drugs contain estrogen and progesteron.

These medicines are used for family planning.

Single large dose is not harmful.

Women often keep oral contraceptives in places where children can easily reach them.

Signs and Symptoms

Nausea and vomiting.

Girls over 4 years of age may have bleeding like a monthly period.

Management

There is no need to do anything. If the patient is a small girl, warn the girl and her parents that she may bleed but that will soon stop.

ORGANOCHLORINES (DDT type Insecticides)

They are widely used as pesticides in agriculture, insect control and malarial control programs.

Symptoms of Toxicity

Nausea, vomiting, confusion, tremors, obtundation, coma seizures and respiratory depression.

Sudden onset of convulsions not preceded by the above premonitory manifestations is a possibility. Sometimes delayed and recurrent seizures can also occur.

Arrhythmia may occur owing to increased myocardial sensitivity to catecholamines.

Management

The clothing should be removed and the whole body sponged or washed with water and soap.

Do not give oil/milk/cream orally.

Emesis is indicated only if patient approaches within 30 minutes of ingestion of organochlorine.

Gastric lavage with lukewarm water or saline is advisable.

Activated charcoal to be given if available.

Supportive measures such as:

Ensure adequate oxygenation and undertake nasophageal suction if necessary.

Give ventilatory support if required.

IV fluids should be given if required—the voulme should be determined by the condition of the patient.

For management of seizures:

Diazepam: Diazepam should be given in undiluted form with close monitoring of blood pressure and respiration.

Followed by either Phenytoin of Phenobarbitone:

Cholestyramine: 4 gms orally is given mixed in fruit juice every 6 hours before meals.

Do not give epinephrine or atropine as these may lead to cardiac arrhythmias.

ORGANOPHOSPHATES (Insecticides)

They are a group of widely used insecticide, pesticides that may cause acute or chronic poisoning. These are used in agriculture, horticulture and also in residences.

Organophosphates
Asenophosmethyl
Carbophenothion
Chlorfenvinphos
Chlorpyritos
Dementon-s-methyl
Diazenin
Dichlorvos
Dimethoate
Disulfolon
Ethoprophos
Fenitrothion
Fonofos
Formothion
Heptenophos
Malathion
Mephosfolan
Mevinphos
Omethoate
Oxydemeton-methyl
Phorate
Phosalone
Phoxin
Pirimyshos methyl
Pyrazophos
Quinalphos
Triazophos
Trichlorphon
Vanidothrin.

These drugs are easily available in the house, are often used for suicidal purposes and are particularly common in developing countries. Accidental poisoning occurs when vegetables and other foodstuffs become contaminated. Accidental poisoning also occurs in individuals involved in spraying these insecticides if proper precatuions are not taken by the handler. Poisoning by inhalation and through contamination is also possible.

Some of the organophosphate compounds are directly toxic while others like malathion and parathion need to be activated in the body.

Following reactions determine the speed of onset and severity of poisoning:

Rate of phosphorylation of the enzyme.

The rate of reactivation of the enzyme through spontaneous hydrolysis.

The rate of ageing of the phosphorylated enzyme by dealkylation. Reactivation is not possible after this step.

LD_{50} of each differs.

Symptoms

Garlic like odour from the patient's breath.

Hyperemia and blisters over the skin at the exposed site.

Inhalation and ingestion may produce local bronchial and gastrointestinal effects, systemic exposure may take longer to develop.

The systemic effects include exaggerated peripheral muscarinic effects, nicotinic actions at neuromuscular junctions and at the sympathatic ganglia.

Mild Poisoning

CNS: Anxiety, restlessness, insomnia, nightmares, tiredness, dizziness, headache.

GIT: Muscarinic effects such as nausea, vomiting, abdominal colic, diarrhoea and tenesmus.

Miscellaneous: Sweating, hypersalivation and tightness in chest.

Moderately, severe poisoning:
Patients show nicotinic effects like muscle fasiculations and generalised skeletal muscle weakness. Patients also experience difficulty in speaking and swallowing.
In severe poisoning:

Consciousness may be impaired. There is flaccid paresis of limbs, respiratory muscles and less often extra-ocular muscles.

Frothy secretions from mouth is a common problem and can embarrass respiration. Pulmonary oedema and cyanosis are also common in severe poisoning.

Atrial fibrillation, heart block and other arrhythmias may occur.

Management

Removal of the patient from contaminated environment. Remove contaminated clothing and wash the exposed skin with water.

Empty stomach by gastric lavage.

Administer activated charcoal.

Collect a blood sample for estimating cholinesterase activity. **However blood cholinesterase levels do not correlate with clinical picture.**

Supportive Treatment

Respiratory secretions should be removed effectively.

Endotracheal intubation is necessary.

Adequacy of ventilation is assessed by doing artrial blood gas analysis.

In case of respiratory depression assisted respiration may be necessary.

In case of vomiting and diarrhoea fluid replacement will be necessary.

In case of subclinical poisoning no treatment is necessary yet patient be kept under observation for about 24 hours. This is done to ensure that delayed toxicity does not develop.

To treat convulsions administer **diazepam** in undiluted form and closely monitor blood pressure and respiration.

Followed by either Phenytoin or Phenobarbitone.

Patient's blood pressure and ECG should be closely monitored.

Atropine is specific antidote

For adults atropine is to be given in the dose of 2 mg IV every 10-30 min till the symptoms subside or signs of atropinisation appear such as flushed dry skin, tachycardia **absence of pulmonary rales** dilated pupils and dry mouth. For children, the required dose of atropine is 0.02 mg/kg but few patients may require upto 0.05 mg/kg. It reduces secretions and reduces bronchospasm.

The duration of therapy depends on clinical status and measurement of cholinesterase activity.

Concurrent administration of pralidoxime and atropine necessitates reduction in the dose of atropine.

When large doses of atropine are given, take care that hypoxia does not develop.

Oximes

Oximes **(Pralindoxime and obedoxime)** are of value if only they are given before the ageing of enzyme occurs. To every symptomatic patient pralidoxme should be given (as it is less toxic than obedoxime) in the dose of 30 mg/kg body weight by slow I.V. injection along with atropine.

The effects of oximes are seen in 30 minutes and include disappearance of seizures, skeletal muscle fasiculations and improvement in muscle power with recovery of consciousness. A further dose of pralidoxime can be given-Pralidoxime mesylate 4 hourly and pralidoxime chloride 6 hourly. In severe cases, repeated doses of pralidoxime may be required for several days.

Diazepam (5-10 mg) controls anxiety but larger doses (10-20 mg I.V.) are required for control of convulsions.

Later neuropathy may be seen.

ORNAMENTAL BEANS (Plant Toxin Irritant)

The beans of plants are made into necklaces and rosaries.

Children are reportedly poisoned by chewing and eating beans from necklaces.

Seeds contain poisons that cause toxicity to blood cells the gut and the kidneys.

The beans can cause death only if they are chewed. Poisoning does not occur if the beans are swallowed whole. Contact with the eyes causes irritation leading to blindness and skin contact may result in a rash.

Signs and Symptoms

If swallowed:

Burning pain in the mouth and throat followed by severe vomiting and pain. Followed by bloody diarrhoea leading to dehydration, drowsiness and convulsions.

Oliguria and haematuria are other features. Blood stained urine is passed in smaller volumes than normal. Death may occur within 14 days.

Management

Take every bit of seed out of the mouth. If the patient has convulsions give diazepam and treat patient symptomatically.

In the Eyes

Wash the eyes for atleast 15-20 minutes with running water.

On the Skin

Wash skin thoroughly with soap and water.

OXALIC ACID (Organic Acid)

In case of Ingestion: Severe burning pain in the mouth, throat, abdomen, dysphagia, gastritis, vomiting, diarrhoea (bloody, mucoid) hypotension with cold clammy skin with rapid pulse. There is metabolic acidosis, hemolysis, massive fluid and electrolyte imbalance (hyperkalemia, hyperphosphatemia, hypocalcemia and hyperchloremia).

In case of Inhalation: Cough, dyspnea, pleuritic chest pain, pulmonary oedema, frothy sputum hemoptysis, bronchospasm, pain in eyes, swelling and lacrimation.

In case of eye exposure: Irritation, pain, lacrimation, swelling, chemosis, photophobia, corneal erosion and perforation, necrosis of conjunctiva and cornea.

In case of dermal exposure: Burning pain, irritation leading to redness, blistering and ulceration.

Management

Same as with other **Acids** *(Refer page 44)*.

OXAMYL (Organophosphorus Compound)

It is an insecticide.

Signs, Symptoms and Management

Same as **Organophosphates** *(Refer page 219)*.

OXAZEPAM (Benzodiazine-Anti Anxiety Agent)

It is benzodiazepine used to treat anxiety.

Symptoms

Mild: Drowsiness, ataxia, weakness.

O

Moderate to severe: Apathy, dizziness, lethargy, slurred speech, partial ptosis, nystagmus, response to verbal stimuli may be intact. Hypotension and respiratory depression.

Management

Often toxicity due to this drug does not require treatment. Gastric lavage is not needed.

Antidote: Symptomatic relief helps. Flumazenil is specific antagonist.

Adult: 0.2 mg over 30 sec. IV repeat at 30 seconds if no recovery occurs repeat dose but total dose should not exceed 3 mg in an hour except in profound coma. Recovery occurs within minutes. If partial recovery occurs increase dose to a maximum of 5 mg. **If no recovery-diagnosis be revised.**

Repeated doses of activated charcoal are recommended only in moderate to severe toxicity.

Ensure adequate oxygenation, provide ventilatory support if required.

IV fluids to be given volume to be determined by the condition of the patient.

Give dopamine if hypotension develops.

Adult: 4-10 ug/kg/min intravenously.

OXYCODONE (A Semisynthetic Opioid)

Signs, Symptoms and Management

Same as with other **Opioids** *(Refer page 215).*

OXYMORPHONE (An Opioid)

Clinical Features and Management

Same as of other **Opioids** *(Refer page 215).*

P

PARACETAMOL (NSAID)

Paracetamol Preparations (Available in India)

Alkasol P, Beserol, Calpol, Cosavil, Crocin, Cyclopam, Dexicat, Febrex plus, Flexon, Metacin, Norfesic, Robinaxol, Sine-Aide, Sudhinol and X-tragesic AF.

Anti-pyretic

It is used as anti-pyretic and analgesic. The anti-inflammatory activity is relatively poor. It does not cause gastritis but is recognised source of toxicity in USA.

Indian figures are not available.

Symptoms of Toxicity

Vomiting is the first symptom and is initially due to drug but subsequently occurs due to liver damage. Patient complains of abdominal pain and tenderness in the right upper quadrant. Between 24-72 hours after ingestion hypoglycemia develops followed by cerebral edema. Between 72-96 hours after ingestion grade 3 encephalopathy develops coupled with abnormalities of liver function tests. After 96 hours of ingestion though prothrombin time improves grade 4 encephalopathy develops and there is brain stem coning. Loss of consciousness normally does not occur.

Hepatotoxicity manifests clinically between 12-36 hours, **enzymes** (SGOT and SGPT) are raised as early as 12 hours. Alkaline phosphatase is minimally raised. Jaundice manifests late.

Rise in bilirubin is slow put prothrombin time gets prolonged within 24-36 hours.

In severe cases if hepatic necrosis is extensive, hepatic failure develops.

Paracetamol also causes **renal tubular necrosis** leading to acute renal failure but is relatively less common than hepatic necrosis. Pain in renal angle associated with albumin urea and haematuria are manifestations of renal involvement. **Plasma creatinine levels are raised before urea.** Though unusual renal failure can occur without hepatic damage.

Hypoglycemia occurs more commonly but in a few patients hyperglycemia may also develop. **Skin rashes, myocardial necrosis and pancreatitis have also been reported.**

High plasma ALT levels > 5000 μ/L is suggestive of paracetamol toxicity as levels of the enzyme to that degree are rarely raised in viral hepatitis.

By the time patient approaches hospital paracetamol disappears from the blood, **therefore blood levels of paracetamol do not aid diagnosis.**

There is high morbidity and mortality if untreated.

Fatal dose is 12 g.

Severity of poisoning is proportional to dose 250 mg/kg produces severe toxicity. **Patients on rifampicin or any other enzyme inducer such as carbamazepine, phenytoin, phenobarbitone or alcohol are at higher risk.**

Management

Specific antidotes—methiomine and N-acetylcysteine.

P **N-acetylcysteine: Complete protection occurs if given within 5 hours of ingestion but efficacy declines drastically if given after 5 hours yet mortality is reduced.**

Dose: 150 mg/kg in 200 ml of 5% dextrose as I/V infusion given over 15 minutes followed by 50 mg/kg in 500 ml of 5% dextrose in 4 hours and then same dose is given for next 8 hours. The last dose is given TDS on the next day.

This is followed by 140 mg/kg orally initially followed by 70 mg/kg four hourly for 17 doses.

N-acetylcysteine produces adverse reactions that are similar to paracetamol. Anaphylactic reactions are also reported.

Methionine: 2.5 gm 4 hourly orally to a total dose of 10 gm.

This is preferred in patients who present early and are suffering from mild to moderate toxicity. Vomiting however may limit its use.

Gastric emptying is indicated only if patient presents within 4 hours and patient has consumed high doses.

Give activated charcoal fresh frozen plasma or clotting factors concentrates along with vitamin K_1 in patients who manifest bleeding tendencies.

Monitor blood glucose along with input/output chart.

Careful control of fluid and electrolytes is essential **Haemodialyses is advocated if patient develops renal failure.**

Phosphatemia needs correcting. Mannitol is given if there is cerebral oedema.

PARA-DICHLOROBENZENE

It is not very toxic amd mild symptoms of gastric irritation may be evident.

Management

Wash chemical off the patients lips. If unconscious and drowsy lay him or her on one side in the recovery position. Check breathing and keep the patient warm.

Ipecac induced emesis is helpful if given early during the course of poisoning.

Do not administer milk, fat or oils which may enhance absorption.

Administer **activated charcoal:**

In case, poisoning occurs in G-6-PD deficient individuals, intravenous hydration and urine alkalization should be done by sodium bicarbonate.

P

PARAQUAT (Herbicide) (Gramoxone)

It is a herbicide used extensively and sold under the name of gramoxone. It is a popular substance for suicidal use in eastern part of the world. It is the active constituent in cleansweep, Dexuron, Famon PD8, Gramazine, Gramonol, Gramoxone, Grounding, Path clear, Scythe, Terraklene, Tota-col and Weedol.

It is sufficiently absorbed from skin to cause serious toxicity. Inhalation on the other hand does not cause serious toxicity.

Solutions are corrosive and this substance produces multiorgan failure with maximum damage to lungs. Importantly **pulmonary toxicity resembles toxicity due to hyperboric oxygen and is worsened by high inspired oxygen tension.**

Symptoms of Toxicity

On inhalation: Sore throat, husky voice and epistaxis are the likely features.

On skin contamination: Can cause fatal toxicity. Features same as on ingestion.

Exposure of eyes: Intense spasm of eyelids, lacrimation and corneal uncleration.

On ingestion: This can occur due to ingestion of crops contaminated with paraquat or attempt at suicide. Corrosive effect is seen in gastro-intestinal tract, along with hepatic necrosis, necrosis of renal tubules and intra-alveolar fibrosis.

On ingestion of 6 gm or more: Nausea, vomiting, abdominal pain and diarrhea occur in about 60 minutes of ingestion.

Hypotension develops both due to fluid loss and myocardial depression.

Metabolic acidosis develops along with convulsions and loss of consciousness.

Between 12-24 hours there is breathlessness, and cyanosis due to pulmonary oedema, resulting in fatal outcome.

On ingestion 3-6 gms of paraquat: Symptoms of gastro-intestinal irritation are of moderate degree, do not result in shock and disappear within a day. However pain in mouth and throat develops producing difficulty in swallowing and speech. Mucus membranes of mouth and tongue become white followed by raw surfaces after 2-3 days. Perforation of esophagus with resultant mediastinitis has been reported. After 72 hours blood chemistry indicates hepato/renal failure. In 5-7 days breathlessness, tachypnoea, crepitations and central cyanosis develop with fatal outcome.

On ingestion of 1.5 to 2.0 gm of paraquat: Nausea, vomiting, diarrhea and mild renal tubular damage. Pain in throat is unusual but ulcerations are uncommon. Breathlessness, basal crepitations and bilateral opacities in X-ray chest are early signs. If untreated, death takes place in 5-6 weeks after ingestion.

Paraquat can be detected in urine. Test: $NaHCO_3$ is added to 5 ml of urine to make it alkaline. Add small amount of sodium dithionate. In presence of paraquat blue colour develops. Degree of colouration is proportional to amount of paraquat. Development of pale green colour in this test indicates very small quantity of paraquat.

Absence of blue colour in urine voided 4 hours after ingestion indicates absence of paraquat ingestion.

Management

Treat skin ulcers as burns. Eyes are washed repeatedly with water.

Activated charcoal needs to be given as early as possible as absorption is rapid. In absence of activated charcoal Fueller's earth (200 ml of a % aquous solution), bentonite (200 ml of a 7% suspension in water and glycerine) can be given gastric lavage is not helpful in reducing absorption.

Haemodialysis is not of much help but charcoal haemo-perfusion is preferable.

Analgesics and anti emetics are given to provide relief from symptoms.

Acetylcystene has been reported to be useful.

For dose of acetylcysteine, see **Paracetamol** *(Refer page 225)*.

PEMOLINE (Amphetamine like)

It is chemically unrelated to amphetamine but clinical picture is same as amphetamine.

It is drug of abuse. It has sympathomimetic activity.

P

Symptoms

Euphoria, talkativeness, restlessness, tachycardia, peripheral vasoconstriction, tachypnea, tremors, dilated pupils may occur along with nausea, vomiting, facial flushing and sweating.

Confusion, delirium, hallucinations, paranoia are prominent.

Serious vascular, cardiac and neurological complications similar to those with cocaine and related products are also seen with this plant.

Hypertension precipitates complications such as dissection of the aorta, myocarditis, myocardial infarction, dilated cardiomyopathy, cerebrospinal fluid rhinorrhoea, subarachnoid haemorrhage, cerebral infarction, cerebral vasculitis, transient cerebral ischaemic attacks, hyperxia, convulsions, metabolic acidosis, impaired consciousness, impaired respiration, and paranoid psychosis.

Management

Administer activated charcoal.

Maintain proper airway.

If conscious is impaired adequate ventilation is necessary. Hypoxia and metabolic acidosis to be corrected if required. Convulsions and agitations are managed by **diazepam.** Hypertension is controlled by **labetolol.**

Labetolol: 0.2-0.3 mg/kg IV or 10-20 mg IV at a rate of 2 mg/min. Further dose is adjusted according to response but maximum dose should not exceed 200 mg.

Beta blockers should be avoided because these cause paradoxical increase in blood pressure. ECG also may show signs of ischaemia because a few beta blockers potentiate coronary vasoconstriction.

Arrhythmias: Extreme tachycardia responds to beta adrenoreceptor blockers which need to be given cautiously and only if necesary. Other cardiac arrhythmias may not be treated unless life threatening.

Forced diuresis can lead to serious trouble in patients with hypertension and arrhythmias.

PENICILLIN

Symptoms

P

Anaphylactic reaction of penicillin is easily confused with following reactions and need differentiating:

a. Procaine reaction is seen after procaine penicillin and is due to procaine and not penicillin. Characteristic features are confusion, hallucinations and psychotic behaviour.

   Symptoms disappear in a short time. Any other salt of penicillin is not likely to produce these features and can be sefely administered.

b. Jasisch-Herxheimer reaction. This reaction occurs in syphelitic patients after first dose of penicillin. This is characterised by chills, fever myalgia and headache. Salicylates can be given to terminate this reaction.

Anaphylactic reaction to penicillin can occur even if patient had received penicillin in the past without allergic manifestations.

Treat symptomatically with adrenaline steroids bronchodilabrs and antihistaminics.

PENTAZOCINE (An Opioid)

Is partial agonist used as analgesic. **Abuse liability is reduced but not absent.**

Pharmacological actions are similar to morphine except that sedation as well as respiratory depression are one-third to half of morphine. More importantly it causes sympathetic stimulation leading to tachycardia and hypertension leading to increase in cardiac load. Thus patients with coronary ischemia and myocardial infarction are at greater risk. **Parenternal administration in morphine addicts precepitates withdrawal.**

Signs and Symptoms of Toxicity

As compared to morphine vomiting is less frequent.

Tachycardia and hypertension are present instead of hypotension sweating and light headedness that may be present initially. High doses produce psychotic behaviour.

Signs and symptoms of acute poisoning usually begin within 20-30 min after oral ingestion and within minutes following parenteral administration.

Shallow breathing with depressed respiratory rate, coma, pin point pupils, cardiac arrhythmias, hypothermia, convulsions, decreased urinary output and gastrointestinal motility-but are less marked than that with morphine. Respiratory depression may lead to hypoxia, cyanosis, bronchospasm, pulmonary edema and respiratory arrest. Deaths are due to respiratory depression and cardiorespiratory arrest.

P

Management

Perform Chemical laboratory analysis of urine blood and a gastric output for presence of drug.

Maintain proper ventilation.
Put an artificial respiration if needed.
IV fluids.

Dopamine: 4-6 ug/kg/min IV.

Gastric lavage.

Activated charcoal: Slurry aqueous or mixed with sorbitol.

Adults dose: 30 to 100 gms.

Children: 10 to 30 gms.

Infant: 1-2 g/kg.

Specific antidote:

Naloxone:

Adult: 1.2 mg I/V.

Children dose: 0.4 to 2.0 mg IV repeat as needed to reverse signs and symptoms of toxicity.

Neonates: Initial dose 10-30 ug/kg IV.

If no response is observed after 10 mg of naloxone have been administered diagnosis of opioid induced poisoning should be questioned.

In responders-continue IV infusion of 2/3 of initial bolus dose of naloxone on hourly basis. Infusion is indicated in poisoning with long acting opioids (methadone). Monitor respiratory rate. CVP carefully during infusion.

Diazepam is given in cases of convulsions:

In adults: 5-10 mg IV initially. Maximum rate 5 mg/min.

Repeat every 10-15 min. Maximum dose 30 mg.

In children: 0.25-0.5 mg/kg IV slowly over 2-3 min.

Repeat every 2-5 min. Maximum dose 5 mg in children below 5 years of age and 10 mg in those above 5 years.

PETROLEUM DISTILLATES

Following are obtained on distillation of petroleum.

Diesel, gasoline, kerosene, naphth, paraffin, petrol and furniture polish.

P

These products differ in chemistry but produce similar toxicity. The above mentioned products are accidentally consumed by children. Kerosene poisoning is quite common in the developing countries as it is used in kitchen for cooking and lighting.

Petroleum distillates are often used as solvent for pesticide and add to toxicity of pesticides.

Symptoms of Toxicity

Vomiting is common but diarrhoea is not a feature.

CNS stimulation leading to excitement and agitation, but in some patients drowsiness is a feature. Convulsions rarely occur.

Pulmonary complications due to aspiration occur in about 60% of cases. Similar pulmonary complications also occur if these products are taken intravenously on ingestion. Pulmonary complications are often seen in patients who fail to vomit after oral intake of distillates. Symptoms associated with lung involvement **(cough, choking, wheezing and breathlessness)** occur within minutes but be delayed by 24 hours.

Central cyanosis may be present. Severe poisoning causes haemorrhagic pulmonary oedema that proves fatal within 24 hours.

Fever and polymorph leukocytosis are commonly associated laboratory findings and are present even in absence of lung involvement. Intravascular haemolysis and renal failure are rare complications.

Double gastric fluid level on X-ray of abdomen in erect posture helps in diagnosis.

Management

If large amount has been consumed gastric lavage is indicated provided patient is fully alert and able to cough. **Olive oil administration reduces absorption of distillates but increases pulmonary problems.**

Hence it is not recommended.

Similarly corticosteroids and antibiotics serve no useful purpose. Antimicrobials are however recommended for patients with secondary bacterial infections. Oxygen is given if patient is cyanosed and intermittent positive pressure respiration given to patients with pulmonary oedema.

PHENCYCLIDINE (Hallucinogen)

P

It is an anticholinergic agent which activates receptors in brain causing disorientation, distortion of body image, hallucination and an anaesthetic state.

Ketamine is closely related compound with lower hallucinogenic potential and is used in anaesthesia.

Management

Ensure that the drug intake is stopped.

All symptoms are reversible and patients recovers.

Gastric lavage: activated charcoal is recommended if high amount has been consumed.

PHENCYLIDINE (Sympathomimetic)

Phencylidine, though produces sympathomimetic activity, does not produce dilation of pupils. On the contrary pupils are small sized and there is multidirectional nystagmus with labile encephalopathy.

Management

Activated charcoal:

Maintain proper airway and provide adequate ventilation Hypoxia and metabolic acidosis to be corrected if required.

Convulsions and agitations are managed by diazepam. Hypertension is controlled by **labetolol**. 10-20 mg IV at a rate of 2 mg/min. Further dose is adjusted according to response but maximum dose should not exceed 200 mg.

Beta blockers should be avoided (except for treating arrhythmias) because these cause paradoxical increase in blood pressure.

Arrhythmias: Extreme tachycardia responds to beta adrenoreceptor blockers. Other cardiac arrhythmias may not be treated unless life threatening.

Forced diuresis should not be produced because forced diuresis can lead to serious trouble in case patient has arrhythmias.

PHENTERMINE (Sympathomimetic Agent)

Phentermine is a sympathomimetic agent. Clinical picture and management same as for **Amphetamine** or **Cocaine** *(Refer pages 57, 92)*.

PHENYL PROPANOLAMINE (Sympathomimetic Agent with Anorexgenic Activity)

P

It is indirectly acting sympathomimetic agent with promiment peripheral effects and less central effects. It is an active principal in nasal decongestant preparations and is often abused for its anorexogenic activity.

Toxicity develops when dose exceeds 75 mg/day.

Symptoms of Toxicity

Nausea, dizziness, nervousness, insomnia, headache, tinnitus, fear, delusions, psychosis and convulsions.

Palpitations and hyperglycemia also reported. Danger is from severe hypertension that is responsible for strokes etc.

Management

Is symptomatic and on similar lines as amphetamine or cocaine *(Refer page 57)*.

PHENYTOIN (Antiepileptic) (Diphenylhydantoin)

Phenytoin is drug of choice for treatment of grandmal seizures, complex partial (temoral lobe; psychomotor seizures and simple partial focal, Jacksonian seizures), but not recommended for pure absence (Petitmal) epilepsy. Parenterally it is given to control status epilepticus of grandmal type. Intravenous preparation is used for treatment of paraxysmal atrial tachycardia, ventricular tachycardia and digitalis induced cardiac arrhythmias.

Large doses are also given for management of trigeminal neuraliga but is less effective than carbamazepine

There are large differences in dissolution rates among various brands, therefore switching over from one preparation to another can cause toxicity.

Symptoms of Toxicity

Oral Toxic Dose: 20 mg/kg (plasma levels >20 ug/ml). Nystagmus, ataxia, slurred speech, ophthalmoplegia hyperreflexia, drowsiness, confusion, disorientation with maniac or hyperactive behaviour. Nausea and vomiting.

On rapid IV infusion (Faster than 50 mg/min): Bradycardia, AV block, hypotension, ventricular fribrillation leading to cardiac decompensation and congestive cardiac failure.

Management

Serum phenytoin concentration is advisable. Therapeutic range is 8-15 mg/l. Any value higher than this indicates impending toxicity.

Gastric lavage:

Adult: 150-200 ml of lukewarm water or saline per wash.

Children: 50-100 ml of normal saline in children below 5 years.

Repeated doses of activated charcoal in normal doses is recommended.

Administer IV fluids, according to the need of the patient.

Blood levels of phenytoin to be monitored so that these do not fall before therapeutic levels and precipitate convulsions.

PHILODENDRON (Plant)

Diffenbactria belongs to the P Araceae family of plants that philodendron and are commonly grown as decorative house plants. Poisoning with this plant is most common in children.

Symptoms

Burning pain in lips and mouth, hypersalivation inflammation of buccal mucosa, lips, tongue and swollen palate.

Respiratory obstruction, retrosternal pain and oesophageal necrosis.

Management

Required treatment is symptomatic.

Advised patient to suck ice and milk.

To treat hyperacidity antacid to be started.

Ranitidine:

Adult: 50 mg IV 6-8 hourly.

Children: 1.25-2 mg/kg/d dose maximum should not exceed 300 mg/day.

In serious respiratory obstruction perform endotracheal intubation (if possible) or tracheostomy.

Corticosteroids: May be given but their value in reducing the oedema has not been assessed.

PHOLCODINE (An Opioid)

Clinical Picture and Management

P

Same as with other **Opioids** *(Refer page 215).*

PHOSPHORIC ACID (ORGANIC ACID)

Symptoms

In case of ingestion: Severe burning pain in the mouth, throat, abdomen, dysphagia, gastritis, vomiting and diarrhoea (bloody, mucoid).

CNS: Hypotension with cold clammy skin and rapid pulse.

Miscellaneous: Metabolic acidosis, hemolysis, massive fluid and electrolyte shifts (hyperkalemia, hyperphosphatemia, hypocalcemia and hyperchloremia).

In case if acid is inhaled: Cough, bronchospasm, dyspnea, pleuritic chest pain, pulmonary oedema, frothy sputum, haemoptysis.

In case of exposure of eyes to acid: Irritation, pain, lacrimation, swelling, chemosis, photophobia, corneal erosion and perforation, necrosis of conjunctiva and cornea.

On dermal exposure: Burning pain, irritation, redness, blistering and ulceration.

Management

In case of inhalation: Patient should be removed from site of exposure and shifted to fresh air.

In case of eye exposure: Depending upon severity irrigate eyes with large volumes of 0.9% normal saline or water for 15 minutes or more.

Wash affected skin with copious amounts of water or mild soap solution.

In case of Ingestion:

Avoid inducing vomiting, Avoid gastric lavage.

Administer water or milk, so that acid can be diluted.

Administer 100% humified oxygen for inhalation. Use respirator if available and necessary.

IV fluids—The volume should be determined by the condition of the patient.

Vasopressors can be used if necessary.

Endoscopy should be done within first 24 hours to determine any kind of perforation along with chest X-ray for detection of mediastinitis or GI perforation.

Antibiotics should be given if perforation is present.

Perform surgery if there is perforation.

Monitor ECG, serum Ca^{++}. If there is evidence of hypocalcemia or severe hypokalemia, administer calcium gluconate (10%) 2-4 ml/kg IV. For topical exposure apply gel containing calcium gluconate (2.5 g/100 ml lubricant).

Precautions

Avoid excessive amount of milk or water as they provoke vomiting.

Avoid carbonated beverages or bicarbonate for neutralization of acid.

P

PLUMBAGO ZLYLANICA (Chitra) and PLUMBAGO ROSEA (Lalchitra) PLANT POISON

Roots of this plant contain a glycoside—The active principal has irritant and narcotic activities (after absorption). It is used to cause abortion or produce artificial bruising.

Symptoms of Toxicity

Pain in stomach, vomiting, thirst and diarrhoea. It is an abortifacient.

Local application produces bruising.

Management

Gastric lavage is given to remove unabsorbed portion of the poison followed by demulcent drinks.

Morphine is given to relieve pain. Hypotension is treated by administering dopamine.

POTASSIUM CARBONATE (Alkali)

Clinical Picture and Management

Same as of other **Alkalies** *(Refer page 49)*.

POTASSIUM CYANIDE

Fatal cyanide poisoning is not always instantaneous except in case of inhalation of large amount of fumes. On ingestion of cyanide salts death occurs after several minutes or even hours.

If source of cyanide is old, death may not occur as cyanide gets converted to hydroxide or carbonate salts.

P

Cyanide is normal constituent of blood of many healthy individuals—though in traces. Vitamin B_{12} and environmental factors such as smoking and eating certain foods contribute to this cyanide.

Ability of individuals to perceive cyanide in bitter almonds is genetically determined. 20-40% human population (mostly males) do not possess this capacity. **Rate of detoxification of cyanide to thiocyanate is also genetically determined.**

Thus patients who lack genetic trait to detoxity cyanide—Leber's hereditary optic atrophy—suffer from optic atrophy.

Management

Perform gastric lavage with 5% solution of sodium thiosulphate. Leave 200 ml of 25% sodium thiosulphate in stomach at the end of lavage.

Maintain clear airway and administer oxygen in high concentrations.

Correct acidosis if present. Improve BP but avoid vasopressors as these are likely to cause arrhythmias.

Patients suffering from low toxicity recover with supportive treatment.

Antidote is given only to treat moderate/severe toxicity e.g. if patient is unconscious.

Dicobalt edetate is antidote of choice—600 mg is given I/V followed by 300 mg I/V after a few minutes (if first dose does not produce appreciable effect). Total dose can be followed by 25 g of glucose I/V.

Alternatively in absence of dicobalt edetate sodium nitrite can be given—10 ml of 3% solution given over 3 minutes.

Sodium thiosulphate—50 ml of 25% solution I/V slowly given over 10 minutes to be given after sodium nitrate.

Pediatric doses: Sodium nitrite 10 mg/kg followed by 5 mg/kg I/V (if necessary).

POTASSIUM HYDROXIDE (Alkali)

Clinical Picture and Management

Same as of other **Alkalies** *(Refer page 49).*

POTATO (SALANUM TUBERCOSUM)

P

It is a common food item. Stem and leaves are toxic. Active principle is an alkaloid—**solanine** which is not normally present in potato. It is present in green potato, or if potatoes have been stored under adverse conditions or if potato is cut and left exposed. **Toxic principle is distroyed on peeling and boiling of potato.**

Poisoning occurs if uncooked/undercooked potato is consumed along with peel.

Symptoms

Vomiting, diarrhea, fever, confusion and delirium with hallucinations and visual blurring.

Death is rare.

Management

Decontamination of gut and supportive measures.

PROPOFOL (Anaesthetic)

It is used intravenously for induction and maintenance of anaesthesia specially for short procedures for outpatient surgery. It crosses placenta and is not recommended for cesarean section.

Symptoms

Causes hypotension-severe in hypovolumic and elderly patients. Causes upper airway obstruction, apnea, hypo-ventilation and despnoea. Convulsions and opisthotonus are also associated with this drug.

Management

Symptomatic treatment is required.

PTOMAINES (FOOD POISONING)

Ptomaines are alkaloids formed due to bacterial de-composition of proteins. In dead bodies these are called cadaveric alkaloid while in living tissues these are referred to as leucomaines. Leucomaines are harmless on ingestion but toxic if administered parenterally.

All ptomaines formed when food is grossly decomposed are harmless except neurine and mydaline. Food poisoning due to these alkaloids causes.

Symptoms resembling atropine and aconite poisoning.

Management is symptomatic.

P

PYRILAMINE (ANTI HISTAMINIC-H_1)

It is an H_1 blocker used to treat allergy, travel sickness and cough. It is often kept in home in places where children can easily get hold of it. As a result, its toxicity is common among children.

Signs and Symptoms

Acute intoxication results in symptoms very similiar to those of anticholinergic poisoning.

Management

Same as for other **Anticholinergic/antihistaminergic agents** *(Refer page 61)*.

Q

QUINALPHOS (Organophosphorins Compound)

It belongs to organophosphorus group of widely used pesticides that may cause acute or chronic poisoning. It is a moderately toxic organophosphorus compound with a LD_{50} of 71mg/kg.

Clinical Picture and Management

Same as for other **Organophosphates** *(Refer page 219)*.

QUINIDINE (Antiarrhythmic Agent)

It is type 1a antiarrhythmic agent and at high concentration reduces myocardial contractility and excitability with severe depression of cardiac conduction velocity. Repolarization is delayed resulting in a prolonged QT interval associated with polymorphic ventricular tachycardia. In addition, it also has alpha receptor blocking activity and anticholinergic activity.

Toxic dose is 1 gm and serum levels > 2-4 mg/L are considered toxic.

Signs and Symptoms

Cardiac Toxicity

Sinus bradycardia and in severe cases may produce SA arrest, prolongation of PR, QRS and QT intervals.

Polymorphous ventricular tachycardias are a possibility.

Depressed myocardial contractility resulting in hypotension and pulmonary edema.

CNS Toxicity

Dry mouth, dilated pupils and delirium.
Seizures and respiratory arrest.
Coma.

Others:
Nausea, Vomiting, Diarrhoea.

Cinchonism occurs with chronic doses (deafness, ringing in the ear and visual impairment).

Diagnosis is based on history of drug ingestion, positive ECG abnormalities and signs and symptoms.

Management

Administer activated charcoal, if available. **Do not induce emesis as it may percipitate seizures.**

Maintain patent airway. Assisted ventilation with oxygen supplementation may be necessary in some cases.

Treat hypotension by fluid therapy instituted at the rate of 10-20 ml/kg along with dopamine, infuse at the rate of 6-10 µg/kg/min.

For treatment of convulsions: **Diazepam** is given in un-diluted form with close monitoring of blood pressure and respiration.

Followed by either Phenytoin or Phenobarbitone.

Ventricular tachycardia be managed in the following manner:

Liodocainei dose (adults and children)-1 mg/kg IV bolus given over 1 minute duration. This is followed by continuous intravenous infusion of 1-4 mg/min (20-50 µg/kg/min) to maintain serum concentration of 1.5-5 mg/L. A repeat dose (0.5 mg/kg IV) can be given after the initial bolus dose if significant ectopy persists.

Do not use lidocaine in the setting of third-degree atrio-ventricular or intraventricular block.

In place of lidocaine phenytoin can also be used.

Q **Loading dose:** 15-20 mg/kg IV for adults and 1 mg/kg in children. Dose is diluted in 50-150 ml of normal saline and given at the rate of 50 mg/min.

Maintenance dose: 5 mg/kg/day as a single oral dose.

Manage "atypical" or polymorphic ventricular tachycardia using overdrive pacing or isoproterenol–1-10 mcg/min IV

Monitor ECG and other vital signs for a miniumum period of 6 hours.

Specific therapy: **Hypertonic sodium bicarbonate:**

Dose: 1-2 mcg/kg rapid IV bolus and repeat every 5-10 minutes. If no response occurs on impaired conduction or on atrioventricular block, insertion of cardiac pacemaker is recommended.

Quinidine is not removed by hemodialysis.

QUININE (Antimalarial)

Quinine sulphate is widely prescribed drug for the management of chloroquine resistant malaria (*P. falciparum*) and for the prevention of nocturnal cramps. Accidental and deliberate acute over dosage toxicity occurs and term **Cinchonism** is used for describing symptoms of its intoxication.

Signs and Symptoms

Mild Toxicity

Nausea.
Vomiting.

Cinchonism is characterized by tinnitus, deafness, vertigo, headache and visual disturbances.

Severe Toxicity

Visual impairment including blindness may occur. Pupils are dilated.

Ocular effects (occur 9-10 hours after ingestion):

Blurred vision, colour blindness, fixed and dilated pupils.

Fundoscopic examination may reveal retinal artery spasm, disk pallor, and macular edema.

Visual impairment may or may not be permanent.

Ataxia, Convulsions and Respiratory arrest can also occur.

Cardiotoxicity is likely to occur and is characterized by hypotension, prolonged QRS and QT interval, AV block and ventricular arrhythmias.

Hypokalemia, hypoglycemia and hemolysis may also occur.

Management

If the patient is fully awake and is breathing normally and is not vomiting, give repeated doses of acitivated charcoal for 24 hours. This helps, provided it is given within 4 hours of ingestion. Quinine has long half life that is reduced by this technique.

Treat convulsions with **Diazepam** given in undiluted form and closely monitor blood pressure and respiration.

Followed by either Phenytoin or Phenobarbitone.

Treat hypotension

Fluid therapy must be instituted at the rate of 10-20 ml/kg with **Dopamine,** that should be infused at the rate of 2-6 μg/kg/min.

The patient should be continuously monitored for vital signs and ECG for atleast 6 hours after ingestion.

Procedures such as hemodialysis and hemoperfusion are ineffective for rapid elimination of the drug as quinine has extensive tissue distribution.

If there is cardiac toxicity it needs appropriate treatment.

Long term prognosis: Visual impairment (reduction in peripheral fields) lasts for long.

R

RED SQUILL

Symptoms

Nausea, severe, vomiting, abdominal pain, ventricular tachycardia, fibrillation and heart block.

Management

Gastric lavage: Use 150-200 ml of normal saline for every wash and repeat after 6-8 hours if required.

Activated charcoal with cathartic: Administer 30-100 gm of activated charcoal with magnesium sulphate or sorbitol.

Phenytoin is given for treatment of arrhythmia. Administer 200 mg. Maximum dose not to exceed 400 mg a day.

RICINUS COMMUNIS (CASTOR) PLANT

Castor (from which castor oil is derived) belongs to family Euphorbiacae. It is large shrub with greenish red leaves. Shrub bears soft spined brown capsules, each contains 3-molted grey-white seeds.

Oil is extracted from the seeds which is pale yellow, viscid liquid, has faint odour and acrid taste. Oil is used as purgative.

The press cake left after extraction of oil, contains an alkaloid-ricin-which is one of the most poisonous substance known.

Symptoms of Toxicity

Vomiting, diarrhea abdominal pain, haemorrhagic gastritic.

Haemolysis may occur leading to severe anaemia haematuria and renal failure.

Anaphylactic shock may occur in a few individuals.

Fatal dose	5-10 seeds or
orally	1 mg/kg body weight of ricin.

Management

Gastric lavage, followed by activated charcoal and purgative are indicated.

I/V fluids and electrolytes are given to correct dehydration and electrolyte imbalance.

For remaining clinical features proceed symptomatically.

RIFAMPICIN (Anti TB/Leprosy)

It is used to treat tuberculosis and other diseases caused by Mycobacteria. It is used with dapsone to treat laprosy. Poisoning from taking a single large dose reportedly resulted in death, but most patients recover if treated. Some people on long term therapy may develop chronic poisoning. Poisoning is more severe in people who frequently drink large amounts of alcohol or have liver disease.

Signs and Symptoms of Toxicity

Acute Poisoning

Orange red coloured urine, sweat and tears. Interestingly **red colour from skin can be removed by washing.**

Warm skin, itching, sweating and swelling of the face.

Nausea, vomiting and abdominal pain.

Lethargy and unconsciousness.

After 6-10 hours, eyes are jaundiced and convulsions may appear.

Death may occur suddenly.

Chronic Poisoning

Nausea, vomiting, constipation or diarrhoea and abdominal pain.

Skin rash, itching and warm skin.

Influenza like symptoms.

Signs of liver and kidney damage (Raised enzymes and urea).

Management

Stop rifampicin immediately and do gastric lavage.

Activated charcoal is recommended. Convulsions are treated by diazepam in usual doses.

S

SALBUTAMOL (Antiasthmatic-Beta$_1$ Agonist)

Salbutamol is commonly prescribed for treatment of asthma and is often kept where children can easily find it. **Young teenagers sometimes abuse salbutamol because it causes feelings of excitement.** It is given by inhalation and oral route is also available.

Symptoms

Excitement and agitation, hallucinations, convulsions tachycardia and palpitations.

Tremors are frequently noted.

Management

Check for fast pulse or palpitations, make the patient rest until the pulse is normal again.

Beta blockers can be given to control tachycardia if severe but this will precipitate asthma. **β_1 specific blockers** are less prone to produce this problem.

SCORPION STING (Animal Toxicity)

Scorpion sting is common in India. Symptoms depend on degree of envenomation.

Symptoms

In most of the cases patient experiences excruciating pain which lasts a few hours. Local burning, pain, paresthesias spreading to the extremities, restlessness, involuntary shaking and jerking movements, muscular fasciculations, excessive lacrimation, rhinorrhea, salivation, perspiration, nausea, vomiting, abdominal pain, hypertension, tachycardia or bradycardia, cardiac arrhythmias of other types, pulmonary edema, spasm in throat leading to respiratory distress, hypotension, shock, disorientation and convulsions. Death occurs due to pulmonary oedema, cardiovascular collapse, coagulopathies, pancreatitis and renal failure.

Management

Advisable laboratory tests in severe envenomation: ECG, BT and CT. PT to monitor disseminated intravascular coagulation, LFT (SGOT) and renal function tests.

Specific treatment: Clean the wound and administer tetanus prophylaxis. Local anaesthesia (xylocaine) may be given at the site of sting if pain is unbearable. Sedative may be required.

Oxygenation.

IV fluids: 5% dextrose.

Children: 5% dextrose.

Treat hypertension if present with labetalol and **Dopamine** is given if hypotension is there. Systolic BP to be kept above 80-90 mmHg therefore, adjust the dose to desired effect.

Diazepam: To treat convulsions if present.

Adult: 5-10 mg IV slowly over 2-3 min. Maximum dose 30 mg.

Children: 0.25-0.4 mg/kg IV slowly over 2-3 min repeat every 2.5 min.

Metoclopramide to control vomiting.

Adult: 5-10 mg IV maximum dose not more than 30 mg/day.

Children: 0.5-1.0 mg/kg Biv, I.V. not more than 4 mg/day. Specially if children are below 1 year dose should not exceed 0.5 mg/kg.

Hydrocortisone is necessary to control allergic reactions.

S

SEMICARPUS ANACARDIUM (Marking Nut)

This belongs to family Anacardiaceae. The tree bears nut like fruits. The acid juice of the fruit is blackish in colour and is used by washermen *(Dhobis)* to mark clothes.

It is often used by quacks for treatment of syphilis, nervous disorders etc.

Symptoms of Toxicity

Juice is irritant and produces inflammatory response when it comes in contact with skin or viscera.

Ingestion causes severe gastroenteritis, hypotension and delirium but death usually does not occur.

Fatal dose 10 gm.

Management

Symptomatic treatment is recommended.

SENNA (Plant Medicine)

Senna is an irritant purgative also used medically.

Some laxative tablets containing senna look and taste like sweets or chocolates and children may eat them by mistake.

Signs and Symptoms of Toxicity

Diarrhoea, vomiting and abdominal pain.

Pink urine if phenolphthalin is also present in the tablet.

In severe toxicity—Blood in stool.
Low blood pressure.
Tachycardia.
Unconsciousness.

Management

Correction of dehydration and electrolyte imbalance is mainstay of therapy.

It is not necessary to make the patient vomit.

Correct electrolyte in balance and replenish fluids according to the need of the patient. This helps in recovery.

SEWER OR DRAIN GAS

S

It is a mixture of several gases, H_2S being the most important constituent responsible for fatal outcome. Small amounts of CO_2 may also be present.

Accidental poisoning due to drain gases are common in India and other developing countries.

Hydrogen Sulfide

'Stink Bombs' contain hydrogen sulfide that may occasionally cause accidental poisoning of large group.

Though hydrogen sulfide has strong unpleasant smell paradoxically its smell cannot be perceived if its concentration is too high. This is due to paralysis of olfactory nerves leading to insidious exposure resulting in serious toxicity.

Symptoms

If percentage of poisonous material is less or exposure is brief—sense of choking with headache, dizziness, vomiting and extreme muscular weakness.

If percentage is high or exposure is prolonged patient feels asphyxiated. Delirium and convulsions appear.

Management

Remove patient to clean air, give artificial respiration along with O_2 inhalation.

SNAKE BITES

Historically, snakes have been amazing. While Indians worship snakes (though largely restricted to cobra), Christianity blames it.

Snake bites are a common accidental poisoning the world over. In India, the maximum cases occur during monsoon. It is interesting to note that in India, more than 65% of the victims of snake bites visit the traditional healers for treatment. Though many herbal medicines are claimed to be effective in treating snake envenomation, the only accepted therapy to date is anti snake venom serum (ASV). Deaths due to snake bites can be substantially reduced with an adequate timely treatment and with appropriate preventive measures.

Snakes

Of the total of 13 families, poisonous snakes belong to five families or sub families classified depending on the morphology of their fangs. Each of these species has typical geographic distribution. For example, snakes belonging to Elapidae are found all over the world except Europe. Russell viper, the commonest cause of poisonous bites in India, is not found in America. Poisonous snakes can be identified by certain morphological features. They possess elliptic pupils, have well developed long and canalized fangs and single row of posterior ventral scales. Their bites usually result in two fang marks with or without small marks of teeth. **The inter-fang distance indicates the size of the snake.** Non-poisonous snakes generally have round pupils, have several rows of small teeth and a double row of posterior ventral plates. Their bites show number of small teeth marks in a row. However, these generalizations do not apply to coral snakes which are colourful, have black, yellow and red bands, round pupils and very short fangs. Most of the non-poisonous snakes belong to Colurbridae family. **Snake should be handled carefully as even decapitated snakes can bite upto one hour.** Cobra, common krait,

Russell's viper and E. carinatus are common poisonous snakes of India.

Differences between poisonous and non-poisonous snakes

Features	*Poisonous*	*Non-poisonous*
1. Belly scales	Large scales covering entire breadth of the belly of snake	Small scales all over the body or moderately large but not covering entire belly
2. Head scale	Small in vipers but larger in pit vipers, cobra, coral snakes and kraits	Large
3. Fangs	Long and either grooved on like injection needles with hollow inside	Short and solid
4. Tails	Compressed	Not compressed
5. Teeth and bite marks	Two long fangs with or without small marks of teeth seen in bites	Bite produces series of small marks

Factors Affecting Severity of Symptoms due to Snake Bites

The average amount of venom injected at a strike and its lethality varies considerably among different species. The amount of venom injected per bite shows a diurnal and seasonable variation. **Bites inflicted at night and immediately after hibernation are the most severe.** There is correlation between the lethality and evolutionary status of a given snake—the more evolved the snake is—the more lethal proved to be its venom. LD_{50} estimations of snake venoms are presented in Table 1 to provide an immediate access to all important venom toxicities.

S

Table 1: Important parameters of some snakes venoms

Snake	*Average length of adults (inches)*	*Dry venom yield (mg)*	*LD_{50} (mg/kg)*
Indian cobra (N naja)	45-65	170-325	0.40
Common krait (B ceruleus)	36-48	8-20	0.09
Russell's viper (V russellii)	40-50	130-250	0.08
Malayan pit viper (A rhodostoma)	25-35	40-60	6.20
Eastern green mamba (D angustceps)	50-72	60-95	0.45
Tiger snake (N scutatus)	30-56	30-70	0.04
European viper (V berus)	18-24	6-18	0.55

Contd...

Contd...

Snake	*Average length of adults (inches)*	*Dry venom yield (mg)*	*LD_{50} (mg/kg)*
Beaked sea snake	30-48	7-20	0.01
Cottonmouth (A piscivorous)	30-50	90-148	4.00
Copperhead (A contortrix)	24-36	40-72	10.50
Tropical rattlesnakes (C devissus terrificus)	20-48	20-40	0.30
Western diamondback (C atrox)	30-65	175-325	3.71

The size of the snake can be approximately determined by noting interfang distance (< 8 mm—small size; 8-12 —medium size; > 12 mm—large size). Larger the snake, higher the quantity of the venom in its glands. **Clinical outcome also depends on the degree of bacterial contamination of the wound** (both of the skin and mouth of the snake). Clostredia and other anaerobes are important contaminants of the wound. As the venom glands do not open at the tip of the fangs, bites which are too superficial are less likely to be envenomated. Various other factors determining the severity are presented in Table 2.

Table 2: Factors affecting the severity of snake bites

1. Severity is proportional to the size of the snake (the larger, injects more poison), the extent of anger, fear or hunger of the snake, condition of its fangs, and amount of venom in the glands.
2. Bites over the face, trunk, or into a blood vessel are more dangerous than bites on limbs or into adipose tissue.
3. Longer the time snake holds on to the bitten area, number of bites it inflicts and deeper the wound, greater will be the toxicity.
4. Presence of bacteria (e.g. Clostredia) in the mouth of the snake and over the bitten part.
5. Children are usually severely increases severity affected due to small body size relative to the amount of venom.
6. Exercise or exertion (e.g. running) speeds up the absorption of the venom and increases the severity.
7. Victim's sensitivity to venom is variable and unpredictable.
8. Last but not the least, the clinical outcome will also depend upon the type of first aid given, the time interval between the bite and medical care rendered.

Clinical Features

Bites from poisonous snakes may result in no injury, local

injury or local injury associated with systemic manifestations. Local pain is not of much help in determining the type of envenomation. Clinical features vary with snake bites with the given species and geographic locations. The characteristic features of major snake groups are given below. After Russell's viper bite, rhabdomyonecrosis and neurotoxicity is predominately seen in Sri Lanka and South India while conjunctival oedema is unique to Burma. The regional variation in features may be because of the differences in the composition of the venom. Many aberrant presentations have also been reported.

A sea snake bite victim presented with pain at local site, regional lymphadenopathy without muscle pain or tenderness which is contrary to the common description. Reynaud's phenomenon and gangrene has been observed in a limb other than that bitten by Russell's viper. Though these are unusual such possibilities should be kept in mind. A frightening response is commonly seen after snake bites.

Specific Features

Elapid bites: At least 50-60% of the patients bitten by elapid snakes do not develop local or systemic features of envenomation. Fangs of elapid snakes are small and thin and hence their marks may not be seen. Pain is an inconstant feature of this envenomation. However, **cobra bites are painful and may be accompanied by local necrosis and sloughing.** Swelling is usual after cobra bite and occurs after a latent period of 15 min to 8 hours. The speed of development and the degree of swelling is comparatively less than after viper bites. **Vomiting, headache, hypotension, drowsiness and polymorphonuclear leukocytosis are suggestive of envenomation.** Numbness and weakness may begin in the region of the bite followed by ataxia, ptosis, glossopharyngeal palsy, pupillary dilatation, slurring of speech and ECG changes. **Increase in cardiac enzymes may be seen.** There is a danger of respiratory paralysis. Muscle paralysis is not a common sequela to cobra bites. If it occurs, it shows early occurrence and rapid progress. Cobra venom can injure visual system by damaging retinal cells, causing bilateral optic neuritis and cortical blindness.

Viper bites: In case of viper bites, **severe local burning pain and swelling starts within a few minutes and gradually spreads. Vomiting, hypotension and signs of abnormal bleeding are early signs of systemic poisoning.** Later features include local swelling and blister formation which may spread. **Low-grade jaundice, pupillary constriction, delirium, convulsions and shock may be seen.** Haemorrhage into a vital organ can occur upto a week after the bite, if no antivenom has been given. **Features may be complicated by secondary infections, acute renal failure, DIC and shock.**

Sea Snake bites: Bites of sea snakes are **painless and without local oedema.** In mild cases, myalgic features may be present which may persist for 1-3 days. **Serum AST is elevated.** In severe cases, symptoms usually begin within 2 hours after the bite. Along with myalgic features, episodic vomiting, sweating and headache soon begin. Passive movements of the body become painful. Generalized muscle pain, weakness, myoglobinuria (after 3-5 hours), ptosis, limb paresis may be seen. Respiratory paralysis may follow. **Hyperkalemia resulting in cardiac arrest and renal failure may occur.**

Complications of snake bites are generally extensions of their pathophysiological features. In India, about 14% of acute renal cortical necrosis cases are caused by snake bites. Along with venom, certain microbes which normally inhabit snake mouth also enter the wound. Rare and unexpected complications are also possible. A rare case of hysterical paralysis is also reported after snake bite. **Snake bites pose a special risk in pregnancy with reported foetal wastage of about 43% and maternal mortality rate of 10% after Crotalidae bite.** Bleeding diathesis can be seen after pit viper poisoning.

Laboratory Features

Relevant history and clinical features are the mainstay of diagnosis. Immunological tests are of benefit in identifying specific snake venom antigens (ELISA). Specific venom detecting kits are now available in certain areas of world. It helps in guiding the therapy if specific antivenoms are available. ELISA is also used in epidemiological studies based on the development and persistence of specific venom antibody. Studies are in progress for the development of a rapid immunoassay technique which can detect the species within 5-10 minutes. In severe cases of poisoning—findings include—progressive anaemia, leukocytosis, thrombocytopenia, hypofibrinogenaemia (resulting in coagulation defects), proteinuria and azotemia. **A negative correlation between serum cholesterol and snake bites of vipera genus has been observed. It may be useful in assessing the severity of these bites.** EEG changes which appear early have been observed in a significant percentage of venomous snake bite cases. The changes were seen mainly in the temporal lobe. However, EEG changes were not correlated with the degree of local swelling or the clinical severity.

Management

First aid measures: Reassure the patient with a view to avoid exertion and vagal effects. Patient should be placed at rest and bitten part immobilized by splinting and placed below the level of the heart (this helps in reducing absorption).

Constriction band: A wide constriction band, if anatomically feasible, made tight enough to allow one finger to pass beneath with moderate resistance, is applied a few cms above the site of bite or the upper limit of the oedema caused by the bite. Constriction band is applied only to impede the lymph flow without obstructing venous flow. This is a potential; dangerous procedure if applied tightly inappropriately as it can result in gangrene, fibrinolysis, peripheral nerve palsy etc.

Emergency Hospital Care

Patients judged as having non-poisonous snake bite should receive antitetanus prophylaxis and antibiotic prophylaxis (cephalosporin is usually indicated) awaiting culture reports. Patient in whom judgement cannot be made as to the poisonousness of the snake should be admitted for constant monitoring (wound as well as systemic symptoms) for at least 8 hours. Mild envenomation requires at least 24 hours of observation in the hospital. Patients bitten by a poisonous snake should be treated as follows:

Admit and carry out baseline investigations, (complete blood count, blood sugar, coagulation screening, blood grouping and cross matching, serum electrolytes, BUN and urine analysis). Keep patient in a quiet environment and reassured.

If necessary, wide constriction band can be applied as described above to delay the absorption of venom. If ASV is indicated, tourniquet should be removed after the administration of ASV. In other cases (if ASV is not available or not indicated), it should remain in place for a few hours or can be moved up the limb gradually as the swelling spreads.

Splinting of the bitten part, and positioning it slightly below the level of heart helps in reducing the absorption of venom.

Incision and suction is not routinely indicated. It may be useful only if carried out within 20-25 minutes of the poisonous snake bite. This procedure can reduce only 20% of the venom injected. **This step is not indicated in coral bites.**

The site of bite should be cleansed and then left strictly alone. If necrosis occurs, the slough needs to be removed. **Potassium permanganate packs applied locally may potentiate local necrosis and are not recommended. Avoid puncturing blisters.**

General measures: I/V fluids are given to support vital functions. **Sedation** may be required, if the patient is apprehensive. **Antihistamines** can be given. For relief of pain, salicylates or meperidine can be administered.

Sensitivity testing for horse serum should be undertaken only if ASV is indicated as judged by the clinical features. It is done with 0.05 to 0.1 ml of 1:10 dilution of the therapeutic serum, intradermally. Immediate reaction appears as wheal with or without erythema within 5 to 30 minutes of the test dose. Shorter the interval (between the injection and the appearance of reaction), greater the sensitivity. However, **a negative test does not rule out the possibility of hypersensitivity. If the reaction is positive, the risk has to be weighed against the possible consequences of withholding the ASV.**

Antivenom serum (ASV): Antivenom is the only specific treatment and its use in severe bites is vital. **It should be given only when there is a clear clinical evidence of systemic envenomation.** ASV sera are a lyophilized powder of horse serum. These give most rapid and effective response. However, **it is not advisable to infiltrate the ASV serum locally. All ASV sera can cause severe allergic reactions which may prove fatal.** Precaution should be taken in this regard. **Shelf life of lyophilised horse serum is generally less than five years.** Potency of ASV should be checked before use by making it sure that it is clear and no opaque substances are present. Depending on the severity of symptoms, 20-100 ml of the serum is diluted in 2-3 volumes of isotonic saline, and is then given by slow I/V infusion at the rate of 10-15 drops/min. **Adrenaline 1:1000 should be available at hand to meet any emergency. Immediate reactions (anaphylaxis, shock)** usually occur within 30 minutes. If reactions develop, the drip should be stopped. Steroids and antihistamines can be used to treat allergic reactions to serum. Adrenaline IM (0.5 ml) is given in case steroids fail to show any effect or the reaction is severe. Several doses of adrenaline may be required to treat this condition. Drip can be restarted afterwards with care. **Children require same or even higher dose of ASV as compared to adults.** Serum sickness can develop 5-24 days after the injection of ASV. It can present with malaise, fever, urticaria, lymphadenopathy, edema, arthralgia or occasionally meningismus or peripheral neuritis.

The role of steroids in the treatment of snake bite has not been clearly defined. However, it may be useful in cobra bites.

There is experimental evidence to suggest that neostigmine can reverse paralysis produced by pure cobra neurotoxin. Repeated half hourly intravenous 0.5 mg of neostigmine with atropine brought about a quicker and better response than ASV alone. Adrenaline has been found to be helpful in paralytic cases.

Tracheostomy, artificial respiration, and fasciectomy are undertaken in treatment of severe bites. Skin grafting may be needed subsequently.

Blood products may be required to manage viperid bites.

Prevention

In snake infested regions one should wear long trousers, high shoes, socks as most of the snake bites are inflicted on lower limbs. Most important is to look where one steps or reaches. Snakes should not be disturbed, attacked or cornered. While going to infested areas, emergency kit along with antivenom should be carried. Vaccination as a preventive strategy has been tried at least for the past 40 years. Various toxoids derived from snake venoms have been experimented in both animals and humans. Though results are encouraging, the practicability of such strategies is at present doubtful. **Health education plays an important role in the prevention of snake bites.** People should be educated about the nature of the snake, magnitude of the problem, importance of early treatment, and useful first aid measures.

Conclusions

Despite tremendous progress, snake bites continues to be one of the major causes of morbidity and mortality in India. The common practice of walking barefoot and popular misconceptions still prevail. Prevalence of variety of snake species with their varied venom composition has made monovalent serotherapy difficult. The vaccination strategies have suffered because of the inadequate knowledge of venom composition and their importance.

SODIUM CARBONATE (Alkali)

Symptoms

Local effects: Burns in lips, oral mucosa, upper airway, oesophagus.

On ingestion: Drooling strider vomiting and gastrointestinal bleeding.

In case of inhalation: Oedema of upper airway, dyspnoea, wheezing, pulmonary oedema, pneumonitis and respiratory failure.

Exposure of eyes: Conjunctival irritation, corneal perforation, distortion of cellular membranes, loss of epithelium of cornea, conjunctiva and lens.

Skin exposure: Pain, redness, irritation and full thickness burns may occur.

Management

In case of Ingestion:

Avoid inducing vomiting. Avoid gastric lavage.

Administer water or milk so that acid can be diluted.

In case of inhalation: Patient should be removed from site of exposure and shifted to fresh air.

In case of eye exposure: Depending upon severity, irrigate with large volumes of 0.9% normal saline or water for 15 minutes or more.

Wash affected skin with copious amounts of water or mild soap solution for 6 to 8 hours.

S

In case of airway compromise do endotracheal intubation and give 100% humified oxygen for inhalation. Use respirator if available and if deemed necessary.

Suction should be done using soft nasogastric tube.

Irrigate mouth frequently in patients who are cooperative and conscious.

I.V. fluids—The volume should be determined according to the condition of the patient.

Vasopressors can be used if necessary.

Endoscopy should be performed within first 24 hours to detect absence or presence of perforation.

Chest X-ray for detection of mediastinitis

Administer antibiotics if there is perforation.

Laparotomy should be done in case endoscopy reveals grade B burns (necrosis of oesophagus or stomach or when signs and symptoms of GI perforation are evident at the time of initial presentation).

SODIUM FLUOROACETATE

Symptoms

Symptoms develop after a delay of minutes to several hours—nausea, diarrhoea, apprehension, cardiac dysarrhythmias, seizures, coma, metabolic acidosis, renal failure, agitation and confusion are reported.

Death in sodium fluoroacetate is due to ventricular tachycardia and fibrillation or respiratory failure secondary to pulmonary edema.

Management

Maintain patent airway and assist ventilation if necessary.

Gastric lavage:

Adult: 150-200 ml of lukewarm water/normal saline.

Children: 50-100 ml of lukewarm water/nornal saline.

If convulsions are present treat with anticonvulsants like diazepam or carbamazepine.

IV fluids: Normal saline is administered to increase excretion of absorbed fluoroacetate and to replenish loss.

SODIUM HYDROXIDE (Soda Washing)

Sodium hydroxide is a corrosive agent used as drain, and pipe cleaner. Accidental poisoning is likely in children. It is a strong alkali and penetrates tissues deeply at a rapid rate; producing necrosis **(acids cause coagulation and have less penetrability).**

Symptoms

Local effects: Burns in lips, oral mucosa and in upper airway, oesophagus.

On ingestion: Drooling strider vomiting and gastrointestinal bleeding.

In case of inhalation: Oedema of upper airway, dyspnoea, wheezing, pulmonary oedema, pneumonitis and respiratory failure.

On exposure of eyes: Conjunctival irritation, corneal perforation, distortion of cellular membranes, loss of epithelium of cornea, conjunctiva and lens (because of penetrability).

Skin exposure: Pain, redness, irritation and full thickness burns.

Management

In case of Ingestion: Avoid inducing vomiting.

Administer water or milk so that acid can be diluted.

In case of inhalation: Patient should be removed from site of exposure and shifted to fresh air.

In case of eye exposure: Depending upon severity, irrigate with large volumes of 0.9% normal saline or water for 15 minutes or more.

Remove contact lenses.

Wash affected skin with copious amounts of water or mild soap solution.

In case of airway compromise do endotracheal intubation. Give 100% humified oxygen for inhalation. Use respirator if available and if deemed necessary.

Suction should be done using soft nasogastric tube.

Irrigate mouth frequently in patients who are cooperative and conscious.

IV fluids—The volume should be determined according to the condition of the patient.

Vasopressors can be used if necessary.

Endoscopy should be performed within first 24 hours to detect absence or presence of perforation.

Perform chest X-ray for mediastinitis. Administer antibiotics if there is perforation.

S

STRYCHNINE (Neurotoxic-Spinal Poison)

It was used as rodentricide and is obtained from seeds of Nux vomica. Seed as such is not toxic as it has hard covering. Brucine is other alkaloid of nux vomica but is less toxic. Strychnine is extremely bitter in taste. This is used both by Ayurvedic and Unani systems of medicine.

It is main ingredient for several vermin killers.

Generally the symptoms appear immediately or within 5-10 minutes but may be delayed in some cases. Fatal dose 60-100 mg in adults.

Symptoms of strychnine resemble tetanus and need differentiating.

Features	*Strychnine*	*Tetanus*
History	Of taking bitter substance	No history/or history of injury
Onset	Sudden, rapidly to either recovery or death	Gradual onset. Death occurs after few days
Muscles	Stiffness of lower jaw occurs **after** all muscles become spastic	**Lock jaw is the first** to develop and spasm of skeletal muscles of body occur later

Strychnine is extremely poisonous if swallowed and works very quickly. Small amounts can cause death but recovery occurs if properly treated.

Symptoms of Toxicity

Stiffness of face and neck.

Fear.

Muscle twitching.

Painful fits and muscle spasms lasting 1-2 minutes, occurring every 5-10 minutes.

The eyes bulge.

The patient is usually weak.

Breathing is difficult and may stop when the patient is having fits, the skin is blue.

High temperature.

S

Signs of kidney damage may be present.

CNS symptoms: (with in 15-20 min).

Muscle twitching, extensive spasm, opisthotonus trismus or facial grimacing, seizures followed by medullary paralysis.

Management

Emesis is not indicated.

Gastric lavage with potassium permagnate:

Adult: 150-200 ml of lukewarm water/saline per wash.

Children: (<5 years) 50-100 ml of saline in children.

Activated charcoal: Is helpful.

Adult: 30-100 gm of activated charcoal with water.

Diazepam: (to treat seizure convulsions): 5-10 mg IV slowly over 2-3 minutes maximum rate 5 mg/min repeat every 10-15 min if seizures are not controlled.

Phenobarbital IV is considered antidote.

Administer IV fluids, according to the need of the patient.

SULFURIC ACID (Strong Acid)

It is corrosive and is used in laboratories.

Accidental poisoning may occur due to pippetting. Actual doses are less important than the concentration of acid.

In case of Ingestion: Severe burning pain in the mouth, throat, abdomen, dysphagia, gastritis, vomiting, diarrhoea (bloody, mucoid) hypotension with cold clammy skin and rapid pulse, metabolic acidosis, hemolysis, massive fluid and electrolyte shifts (hyperkalemia, hyperphosphatemia, hypocalcemia and hyperchloremia).

In case of Inhalation: Cough, dyspnea, pleuritic chest pain, pulmonary oedema, frothy sputum, hemoptysis, bronchospasm, pain in eyes, swelling and lacrimation.

In case of eye exposure: Irritation, pain, lacrimation, swelling, chemosis, photophobia, corneal erosion and perforation, necrosis of conjunctiva and cornea.

In case of dermal exposure: Thickness of skin with burning pain, irritation, redness, blistering and ulceration.

Management

In case of Ingestion:

Do not induce vomiting or gastric lavage.

Administer water or milk in order to dilute the poison.

Patient should be shifted to fresh air in case of inhalation.

In case of eye exposure, irrigate with large volumes of 0.9% normal saline or water for 15 minutes or more depending upon severity.

Wash affected skin with copious amounts of water or mild soap solution.

Do not give excessive amount of milk or water as it provokes vomiting.

Do not give carbonated beverages or bicarbonate for neutralization.

Do endotracheal intubation in case of airway compromise and give 100% humified oxygen with assisted ventilation.

Suction should be done by soft nasogastric tube.

Irrigate mouth with water in cooperative patient or intubate unconscious patients.

IV fluids to be given according to need.

Vasopressors are given to correct BP.

Antibiotics if there is suspicion of infection or if there is intestinal perforation.

Peform endoscopy within first 24 hours and chest X-ray for detecting mediastinitis or GI perforation and treat surgically if these are detected.

T

TEMEPHOS (Organophosphorus Compound)

It is organophosphorus compound that is widely used as pesticide that may cause acute or chronic poisoning. It is a relatively less toxic organophosphorus compound with an LD_{50} of 4204-5000 mg/kg.

Clinical Picture and Management

Same as for other **Organophosphorus compounds** *(Refer page 219).*

TERAZOSIN (Vasodilator)

It is a peripheral vasodilator and serious acute overdoses seldom occur.

Minimum toxic levels have not been established.

Clinical Presentation

Headache
Nausea
Dizziness
Weakness
Syncope
Orthostatic hypotension
Warm flushed skin
Palpitation
Lethargy
Ataxia

Severe hypotension may result in cerebral and myocardial ischemia and acute renal failure.

Treatment

Assisted ventilation with oxygen supplementation should be provided if necessary.

Vasodilator overdose induced hypotension usually responds to supine positioning. In case no effect is seen, administer IV fluids with dopamine at the rate of 6-10 µg/kg. **Higher concentration may result in severe peripheral vasoconstriction and gangrene.**

For decontamination, **activated charcoal** without purgative is effective. Gastric emptying is not necessary if activated charcoal is given promptly.

TERFENADINE (ANTIHISTAMINIC H_1)

It is non-sedative antihistaminic was used to treat allergies. The use has declined as it is cardiotoxic.

Symptoms

Drowsiness.

Prolongation of QTc interval.

Ventricular tachycardia.

In some cases **torsade de pointes with or without giant U waves has been seen.**

Management

It is wise to put the patient under observation for atleast 12 hours.

If QT interval prolonged cardiac monitoring is required.

Intravenous magnesium sulphate abolished ventricular ectopic beats and tachycardia in one man.

TETANUS (Infection)

It is a disease caused by an exotoxin produced by Clostridium tetanus, an anaerobic, spore forming, gram-positive rod found widely in soil and in the gastrointestinal tract. Tetanus is typically seen in older persons specially women.

Symptoms

The most common initial complaint is pain and stiffness of the jaw, progressing to trismus, sinus sardonicus and opisthotonus over several days. Uncontrollable and painful reflex spasm involving all muscle groups are precipitated by minimal stimuli and can result in fractures, rhabdomyolysis, hyperpyrexia and asphyxia. The patient remains awake during the spasms. In survivors the spasm may persist for days or weeks.

A syndrome of sympathetic hyperactivity often accompanies the muscular manifestations with hypertension, tachycardia, arrhythmias and diaphoresis.

Cephalic tetanus is often associated with head wounds and involves primarily the cranial nerves.

Management

Prevention can be ensured by complete immunization with tetanus toxoid in childhood and repeated booster doses at 10-year intervals.

Emergency and Supportive Measures

Maintain the airway and assist ventilation if necessary.

Treat hyperthermia, arrhythmias, metabolic acidosis and rhabdomyolysis if they occur.

Minimise external stimuli such as noise, light and touch.

Treat muscle spasms aggressively by:

Administering **diazepam or midazolam** to patients with mild muscle contraction. **Give morphine.**

In more severe case, use skeletal muscle relaxant—**pancuronium**—to produce complete neuro muscular paralysis.

Specific Drugs and Antidotes:

Human tetanus immune globulin (TIG) 3000-5000 is administered IM. This will neutralize circulating toxin but **has no effect on toxin already fixed to neurons.** It should be given as early as possible to a patient with suspected tetanus and to persons with fresh wound but with inadequate immunization.

Thoroughly debride and irrigate the wound and administer appropriate antibiotics.

TETRACHLORVINPHOS (Organophosphorus—Insecticide)

It belongs to organophosphorus group of widely used pesticides that may cause acute or chronic poisoning. It is a relatively less toxic organophosphorus compound with an LD_{50} of 4000-5000 mg/kg.

Clinical Picture and Management

Same as of other **Organophosphates** *(Refer page 219).*

THALLIUM

Salts are used to kill rats, mice and other rodents and ants.

Affects the gut, nerves, skin and hair.

Exposure to small amounts over many weeks, by swallowing or constant skin contact or breathing in metal fumes can cause chronic poisoning.

Special risk groups:

Thallium rat bait made with grain, biscuit or honey may be mistaken for food. Industrial workers may get chronic poisoning from breathing in fumes or dust.

Symptoms

Signs and symptoms appear within 12-24 hours.

Metallic taste, dryness of mouth, soreness of gums, rhinorrhea, conjuctivitis, puffiness of face and eyes, salivation, nausea, vomiting, bloody diarrhoea, hematemesis, abdominal pain that may progressing to small intestinal obstruction.

Symptoms after 2-5 days.

Headache, lethargy, muscle weakness, paresthesias, tremors, ptosis, ataxia, myoclonic movements, psychosis, seizures, delirium and coma.

Symptoms around 7 days:

Pain or numbness in the soles of the feet so that the patient cannot stand or move.
Dizziness.
Drooping eyelids.
Fever.
Jumbled speech and confused behaviour.
Trembling, strange movements of the arms and legs.
Signs of kidney damage. Abnormalities in RFT.

Chronic Poisoning

T

Hair fall out leaving bald patches.
Wet mouth.
Blue line on the gums.
Nausea, vomiting, belly pain and constipation.

Management

No specific antidote is available.
Clear airway by nasopharyngeal suction of secretion/ vomitus.

Administer oxygen, IV fluids: Normal saline 20 ml/kg.

Perform gastric lavage: 150-200 ml lukewarm water/ saline administer with 1% sodium or potassium iodide.

Give **activated charcoal** 70-100 gm.

Potassium chloride infusion 10 mEq is given to displace thallium from cells and this increases excretion of thallium.

If patient is having seizures administer diazepam (5-10 mg/IV) slowly over 2-3 minutes maximum rate is 5 mg/min repeat every 10-15 min if required.

THEOPHYLLINE (Antiasthmatic)

It is a methylxanthine widely used for the treatment of asthma. Intravenous infusions of aminophylline, the ethylenediamine salt of theophylline is used to treat bronchospasm, congestive heart failure and neonatal apnea. Theophylline is most commonly used orally in sustained release preparations.

Symptoms

Usual manifestations include vomiting, tremors, anxiety and tachycardia. Metabolic effects include pronounced hypokalemia, hypophosphatemia, hyperglycemia and metabolic acidosis.

With serum levels above 100 mg/L, hypotension, ventricular arrhythmias and seizures are common. Status epilepticus is frequently resistant to anticonvulsant drugs.

Seizures and other manifestations of severe toxicity may be delayed 12-16 hours or more after ingestion.

Management

Maintain patency of airway and assist ventilation if necessary.

T

Treat seizures with diazepam. Tachyarrhythmias and hypotension are best treated with a beta adrenergic agent.

Hypokalemia usually resolves spontaneously without aggressive treatment.

Monitor vital signs, ECG and serial theophylline levels at least 16-18 hours after a significant oral overdose.

Specific Drugs and Antidotes: Hypotension, tachycardia and ventricular arrhythmias are caused primarily by excessive beta-adrenergic stimulation. Treat with low dose **propranolol or esmolol.**

Administer activated charcoal, if available. Ipecac induced emesis may be useful for initial treatment at the scene.

Gastric emptying is not necessary for small ingestions if activated charcoal can be given promptly.

Undissolved sustained release tablets may not be removed with gastric tube. For massive ingestions following special techniques are required to be undertaken:

Administer repeated doses of activated charcoal.

Perform whole bowel irrigation.

Theophylline has a small volume of distribution and is effectively removed by **dialysis,** charcoal hemoperfusion or repeat dose activated charcoal.

THIOFANOX (Carbamate Insecticide)

Clinical Features

Same as with other **Carbamates** *(Refer page 87).*

Treat like **Organophosphates without oximes** *(Refer page 219).*

THIOMETON

Clinical Features

Same as with other Carbamates *(Refer page 87).*

Treat like **Organophosphates without oximes** *(Refer page 219).*

THIONAZIN (Carbamate)

Clinical Features

Same as with other Carbamates *(Refer page 87).*

Treat like **Organophosphates without oximes** *(Refer page 219).*

T

THYROID HORMONE

In spite of potentially life threatening manifestations of thyrotoxicosis **serious toxicity rarely occurs after acute thyroid hormone ingestion.**

Symptoms

Mild to moderate intoxication may cause sinus tachycardia, elevated body temperature, diarrhoea, vomiting, headache, anxiety, agitation, psychosis and confusion.

Severe toxicity may include supraventricular tachycardia, hyperthermia and hypertension.

TSH is lowered and serum T_4 remains high for 15 days.

Management

Maintain patency of airway and assist ventilation if necessary.

Most patients will suffer no serious toxicity or will recover with simple supportive care as thyroxine has short half life.

Treat serious tachyarrhythmias with propranolol or esmolol.

Administer activated charcoal along with a purgative. Ipecac induced emesis may be useful for initial treatment.

Charcoal hemoperfusion may be effective so can be performed.

TINCTURE OPIUM (Narcotic Drug)

Signs and symptoms of acute poisoning usually begin within 30-40 mins after oral ingestion.

Shallow breathing with depressed respiratory rate, coma, pin point pupils, bradycardia, cardiac arrhythmias, hypotension, hypothermia, convulsions, decreased urinary output and gastrointestinal motility. Respiratory depression may lead to hypoxia, cyanosis, bronchospasm, pulmonary edema and respiratory arrest. Deaths in opioid poisoning are due to respiratory depression and cardiorespiratory arrest.

Manage as **Opioid** *(Refer page 215)*.

T

TOXAPHENE (Organochlorine Insecticide)

It is widely used as a pesticide in agriculture, insect control and malarial control programs. It is moderately toxic among organochlorines with animal oral LD_{50} > 50 mg/kg.

Clinical Picture and Management

Same as of other **Organochlorines** *(Refer page 218)*.

TRANYLCYPROMINE (Antidepressant—MAO Inhibitor)

It is used as an antidepressant and serious toxicity results from overdose or due to interactions with certain other drugs or foods.

Ingestion of even 2-3 mg/kg of the drug may be life threatening. **Because of irreversible inhibition of the enzyme, adverse drug interactions may occur for upto 2 weeks after discontinuing them.**

Symptoms of Toxicity

Even after acute ingestion of the overdose of tranylcypromine, it takes 6-24 hours before symptoms are evident. However, if interacting drug/food is taken in the meantime, symptoms may be precipitated immediately.

Mild Toxicity

Anxiety, Flushing, Headache, Tremors.

Myoclonus, Hyperreflexia, Sweating, Shivering, and Tachypnea.

Moderate hypertension or Orthostatic hypotension—both are possible.

Severe Toxicity

Severe hypertension resulting in intracranial hemorrhage Delirium Hyperthermia.

Cardiovascular collapse and multisystem failure are the cause of death.

Serotonin syndrome is characterized by severe rigidity, hyperthermia myoclonic jerking, hyperreflexia and diaphoresis when patients poisoned with MAO inhibitor consumes one of the following; **meperidine, dextromethorphan, fluoxetine, paroxetine, sertraline, or tryptophan.**

Management

Maintenance of airway and ventilation is important. If deemed necessary, assisted ventilation with oxygen supplementation may be provided.

Treat hypertension by the use of any **one of the following** drugs:

Phentolamine: 1-5 mg IV (children 0.02-0.1 mg/kg) as a bolus, repeat at 5-10 minutes intervals (or constant infusion of 0.1-2 mg/min) as needed to lower blood pressure to a desired level (usually <100 mg/Hg diastolic in adults and 80 mm Hg diastolic in children).

Nifedipine: 10 mg sublingually for adults and 0.25-0.5 mg/kg/dose for children. Do not use extended release formulation for sublingual administration.

Nitroprusside: It should only be used in emergency or intensive care setting. Blood pressure should be monitored continuously or frequently.

T

Dosage: The average dose is 3 μg/kg/min in children and adults and maximum rate should not exceed 10 μg/kg/min to avoid risk of acute cyanide toxicity. For preparation of the intravenous solution, dissolve 50 mg of sodium nitroprusside in 3 ml of 5% dextrose and dilute this solution in 5% dextrose to achieve concentration of 200, 100 or 50 μg/ml respectively. Initiate with 0.3 μg/kg/min and titrate the dose to a desired effect. In case no effect on blood pressure is seen, use an alternative.

Nitroprusside solution is photosensitive and, therefore, the bottle and intravenous tubing should be protected from light.

In case, tachycardia is also present, **add one of the following** to the above mentioned treatment.

Propranolol: 0.02-0.1 mg/kg IV.

Esmolol: 25-100 μ/kg/min IV.

Labetolol: 0.2-0.3 mg/kg IV.

Do not use beta blockers alone for treatment of hypertension as it might result in paradoxical rise in BP.

In case of abnormal neurological findings, a CT scan is advisable to rule out stroke.

Convulsions should be managed by **Diazepam** given in undiluted form with close monitoring of blood pressure and respiration.

Followed by either Phenytoin or phenobarbiturate.

T

Treat hyperthermia by external cooling—the most efficient way of cooling. In case shivering occurs as a consequence of cooling, use diazepam (0.1-0.2 mg/kg IV) or midazolam (0.05-0.1 mg/kg IV) to treat/prevent it.

For treating serotonin syndrome, use diazepam for controlling seizures as described above and apply external cooling.

Continuously monitor temperature, vital signs and ECG for a minimum of 6 hours in asymptomatic patients and admit all symptomatic patients for continuous monitoring.

TRICHLOROETHANE AND TRICHLOROETHYLENE

Are volatilate and inflammable organic solvents mainly used in laboratories and in house typewriter correction fluid (white fliud), colour film cleaners, insecticides, spot removers and paint removers. It can be absorbed through the lungs, skin and alimentary tract. Poisoning in children is common but serious poisoning is rare.

Symptoms

Loss of consciousness, depressed rate of respiration and convulsions are the most common symptoms of toxicity. Both these agents show disulfiram type of reaction with alcohol.

Management

There is no specific treatment.

Patient should be evacuated from the toxic atmosphere. Clothes must be removed and the skin thoroughly washed.

Maintain patent airway and assist respiration if needed.

Treat convulsions by diazepam.

Repeat the diazepam dose every 10-15 min if necessary. Maximum dose—30 mg for adults and 5 mg for children under 5 years and 10 mg for children over 10 years.

Diazepam should be followed by either **Phenytoin or phenobarbitions IV.**

Treat arrhythmias with propranolol (1-2 mg IV) or esmolol (25-100 μg/kg/min IV).

Give activated charcoal and repeat without purgative every 4-6 hours.

Prognosis

Recovery of consciousness may occur within a few hours but glucose tolerance may take few months to return to normal.

T

TRICHLORPHON (Organophosphate Insecticide)

Clinical Features and Management

Same as for other **Organophosphates** *(Refer page 219)*.

TRIMIPRAMINE (Tricyclic Antidepressant)

It is used as **Antidepressant** *(Refer page 58)*.

TRIPELENNAMINE (Anti Histaminic H_1)

It is an H_1 blocker used to treat allergy, travel sickness and cough. It is often kept in home in places where children can easily get hold of it. As a result, its toxicity is common among children.

Clinical Picture and Management

Same as other **Antihistaminics** *(Refer page 61)*.

TURPENTINE (Petroleum Distillate)

Clinical Picture and Management

Same as **Petroleum distillates** *(Refer page 232)*.

Turpentine comprises mixture of pinene, camphenes, and other terpenes. Accidental ingestion by children is common.

TURPENTINE SUBSTITUTE (White Spirit)

Turpentine substitute (White spirit) is a mixture of long chain hydrocarbons that is used as point thinner.

Clinical Picture and Management

Same as for **Petroleum distillates** *(Refer page 232)*.

U

URAPIDIL (Vasodilator)

It is a peripheral vasodilator and serious acute overdoses seldom occurs.

Toxic levels: Minimum toxic levels have not been established.

Clinical Presentation

Headache, Nausea, Dizziness, Weakness, Syncope, Orthostatic hypotension and Ataxia.

Warm flushed skin and palpitations.

Lethargy.

Severe hypotension may result in cerebral and myocardial ischemia and acute renal failure.

Management

Assisted ventilation with oxygen supplementation should be provided if it is necessary.

Vasodilator overdose induced hypotension mostly responds to supine positioning. In case no effect is seen, fluid therapy must be instituted at the rate of 10-20 ml/kg.

Add dopamine. Infuse 4-6 μg/kg/min. Higher doses may result in severe peripheral vasoconstriction and gangrene and should be avoided.

For decontamination, activated charcoal is effective. Gastric emptying is not necessary if activated charcoal is given promptly.

V

VALPROATE SODIUM (Antiepileptic)

It is broad spectrum antiepileptic agent. Is drug of choice for management of absence seizures. Atypical absence seizures and myoclonic epilepsy respond to this drug. It is also used for treatment of bipolar disorder and in treatment of aggression or violence.

Symptoms of Toxicity

Weight gain (11%) on prolonged use.

Sedation, nausea, headache tremors, hair loss and dizziness.

Rarely skin rashes, enuresis, insomnia, anxiety, fatigue and paraesthesias are also observed.

Heaptic failure is common in patients on polytherapy and in children.

Death occurs due to hepatic failure and CNS depression.

Management

Symptomatic therapy is recommended.

VAMIDOTHION (Organophosphorus Compound)

Clinical Features and Management

Same as with other **Organophosphorus compounds** *(Refer page 219)*.

VASODILATORS (Diazoxide, Doxazosin, Hydralazine, Indoramin, Minoxidil, Phenoxybenzamine, Phentolamine, Prazosin, Terazosin and Urapidil)

Various vasodilators and alpha blockers are used as antihypertensives in clinical medicine. Although, serious toxicity does not occur in adults, coma may occur in the elderly patients.

Toxic: Minimum toxic levels have not been established.

Clinical Symptoms

Headache, Nausea, Dizziness, Weakness, Syncope, Orthostatic hypotension and Ataxia.

Warm flushed skin and palpitations.

Lethargy.

Severe hypotension may result in cerebral and myocardial ischemia and acute renal failure.

Management

Assisted ventilation with oxygen supplementation should be provided if it is necessary.

Vasodilator overdose induced hypotension mostly responds to supine positioning. In case no effect is seen, fluid therapy must be instituted at the rate of 10-20 ml/kg.

Add dopamine. Infuse 4-6 μg/kg/min. Higher doses may result in severe peripheral vasoconstriction and gangrene and should be avoided.

For decontamination, activated charcoal is effective. Gastric emptying is not necessary if activated charcoal is given promptly.

VOLATILE SUBSTANCE ABUSE—Acetone, Butane, Carbon Tetrachloride, Chloroform, Ether, Fluorinated hydrocarbons, n-hexane paraffin hydrocarbons, Methylene chloride, Petrol, Tetrachloroethylene, Toluene, Trichloroethane and Trichloraethylene.

The above substances are inhaled for pleasurable effects. These are also referred to as solvent abuse e.g. glue snuffing or solvent sniffing.

Combination of these substances are available in polishes, spot and nail polish removers, dry cleaning agents, paint thinners, fire extinguishers and antifreeze preparations.

All the above mentioned substances in small doses cause CNS stimulation while longer inhalations of concentrated product produces CNS depression.

Symptoms of Toxicity

There is CNS excitement leading to sense of well-being that may be accompanied by hallucinations. These symptoms are followed by dizziness, ataxia, sneezing and coughing (due to irritation of respiratory tract).

Higher dose causes impairment of consciousness/ mental confusion, loss of self control, dysarthria and nystagmus. Convulsions may occur due to hypoxia followed by coma.

If these are combined with halogenated hydrocarbons (e.g. Chloroform) or beta agonists (e.g. Anti-asthmatic) cardiac arrhythmias may develop leading to fatal outcome. Severe metabolic acidosis may occur.

Sniffers usually seek medical help for late complications such as jaundice and renal damage that are often seen in toluene or carbon tetrachloride users.

Chronic encephalopathy is seen in users of petrol with high tetraethyl load (not with deleaded petrol) and mixed polyneuropathy with hexane.

Premature labour, perinatal deaths and fetal growth retardation results if these products are snuffed during pregnancy.

Management

Stop snuffing and keep the patient away from the contaminated environment.

Sedation may be given during period of excitement. Correct acidosis (if present) by administering sodium bicarbonate.

In case of heavy exposure to carbon tetrachloride. N-acetyl cysteine150 mg per kg body weight dissolved in 200 ml of 5% dextrose is given in 15 minutes followed by 50 mg/ kg body weight in 500 ml of 5% dextrose as I/V infusion in 4 hours and then the same dose is given for next 8 hours.

On the following day 50 mg/kg acetylcysteine in 5% dextrose (500 ml) is given three times I/V. Administration is followed by 140 mg/kg oral dose of acetylcysteine followed by 17 doses of 70 mg/kg given every four hourly.

N-acetylcysteine may produce, flushing, urticaria, angioedema, respiratory distress along with hypotension. However these are rare and disappear on discontinuation of drip. In such patients drug can be restarted at a slower rate. If serious reactions occur antihistamine is recommended.

W

WARFARIN AND SUPERWARFARINS (Oral Anticoagulants-Brodifacoum, Bromadrolone chlorphaninone coumatetralyul, Defencoum Flocobdmafen. All are rodenticides)

These substances are used as rodenticides.

Symptoms of Toxicity

With ingestion of long acting preparations: Bruising, bleeding from nose, gums, haematuria and menorrhagia. Other symptoms include backache, bleeding lips and mucus, membranes, hemorrhage, abdominal pain, vomiting and petechial rash. Later-paralysis may occur due to cerebral hemorrhage shock and death may occur.

Children can easily access the rat poison as these are kept open specially if not stored properly.

Management

Swallowing a small amount of these agent does not lead to poisoning.

Gastric lavage should be avoided in warfarin but advised in superwarfarin.

Cholestyramine 4 gms is given orally in fruit juice every 6 hours before meals. Cholestyramine orally enhances elimination of warfarin in stools.

Parenteral vitamin K_1 IV 60 mg/day along with infusion of fresh frozen plasma (if patient has bled).

Monitor prothrombin time and keep it between 2-3 times the normal.

WATER HEMLOCK (Plant Toxin)

Water hemlock and hemlock water drop wart belong to Umbethferace family of poisonous plants. Poisoning usually occurs due to ingestion of the roots, little rhizome of water hemlock may be fatal for an adult.

Symptoms of Toxicity

Symptoms one hour after ingestion:

Malaise, nausea, hypersalivation, vomiting, abdominal cramps, extensor muscle spasm, opisthotonous, convulsions, dilated pupils, cyanosis, pyrexia, either bradycardia or tachycardia, parotid gland enlargement, flushing of the skin, leukocytosis, metabolic acidosis, elevated serum phosphokinase, elevated aminotransferase, toxic myositis, jaundice and hypoprothrombinaemia.

Management

No specific treatment is available. The stomach should be emptied.

Diazepam: (If convulsions present).

Adult: 5-10 mg intravenously slowly over a period of 2-3 minutes. **Child:** 0.25-0.4 mg/kg intravenous slowly over a period of 2-3 min.

Dantrolene : (If muscle tone is increased) 1-2 mg/kg IV rapidly, may be repeated as needed every 5-10 minutes to a total dose of 10 mg/kg. Give 1-2 mg/kg IV or orally upto maximum of 100 mg 4 times a day for 2-3 days to prevent recurrence of hyperthermia.

Other symptoms should be treated symptomatically and conventionally.

WOOD ALCOHOL (Methanol, Methylalcohol)

Same as with other **Methanol** *(Refer page 186)*.

WASPS

Of various types of wasps, yellow jackets are most aggressive and sting without provocation. Other wasps are non-aggressive and sting only if their life is disturbed.

W

Stinger of wasps does not have barbs and can easily be withdrawn. Multiple stings are common. Wasp venom contains dopamine, histamine, serotonin and some time acetylcholine and vasoactive kinins.

Symptoms

Local irritation and pain.

In addition can cause infection during a sting. Cellulition may result.

Management

Symptomatic treatment given.

Antibiotics are recommended for prophylaxis.

Y

YELLOW OLEANDER (Cerebra Thevatia)

Seeds of this plant are toxic. The active principles are—**Thevetm and Cerberin.**

One fruit contains one nut and one nut contains two karnels. 8-10 seeds (kernels) prove fatal.

Symptoms of Toxicity

Burning sensation in mouth and dryness of throat with tingling sensation. Patient experiences headache, giddiness and feeling of faintness. Pupils are dilated while the skin is cold and clammy. Pulse is weak, irregular, slow and of low volume.

Both vomiting and diarrhoea are likely to be present.

Patient may experience tetanic convulsions.

Management

Gastric lavage is useful if carried out early.

Sodium lactate is given I/V to combat acidosis.

5% glucose with 1.2 mg atropine along with 2 ml of adrenaline is given if there is marked bradycardia and hypotension.

YELLOW PHOSPHORUS

White or Yellow Phosphorus

It is white or yellowish in colour with garlic odour. It ignites at 34°C and produces white fumes. It is used in fireworks, gunpowder preparations also in fertilisers, vermin paste and as rodenticide.

It is protoplasmic poison and affects cellular oxidation. It is commercially used to make verminpaste—that is composed of white arsenic, yellow phosphorus (to keep it glowing at night) and prussian blue or indigo to attract ants during the day.

It is not used on match sticks.

Tip of safety match stick consists of combination of potassium chlorate or lead oxide or potassium dichromate, antimony disulphide and either powdered glass or coarse particles of sand. The ignitor surface (box surface) of match box contains red phosphorus (non toxic), coarse sand and glue.

Red phosphorus *per se* is non toxic but commercially available red phosphorus is toxic as it contains 6% yellow phosphorus.

Phosphorus poisoning is not common in India.

Symptoms

In yellow phosphorus toxicity symptoms due to ingestion occur in three phases.

Phase I (just after ingestion): Garlic like smell in breath, burning pain in the throat, chest and abdomen, nausea, vomiting, diarrhoea and smoky stools with headache and seizures.

Phase II: In this phase no symptoms are present.

Phase III: Hepatic and renal failure, shock, diathesis and encephalopathy. Death in case of yellow phosphorus is due to cardiovascular collapse.

On skin contamination: Second and third degree burns.

Management

IV fluids.

Gastric lavage with either potassium permagnate or hydrogen peroxide: 150-200 ml of lukewarm water/saline for every wash with potassium permagnate (1:5000 conc.) or with 2% hydrogen peroxide.

Diazepam (If patient has convulsions): 5-10 mg IV slowly every 2-3 min. Maximum rate 5 mg/min. Repeat every 10-15 min if required. Dose should not exceed 30 mg.

Or

Y

Phenytoin: To treat convulsions.

Adult: 10-15 mg/kg by slow IV injection. Maximum rate 5 mg/min. 100 mg orally or IV every 6-8 hours.

Children: 15-20 mg/kg IV slowly at the rate of 1 mg/kg/min 1.5 mg/kg every 30 min. Maximum dose 20 mg/kg/day.

YEW (Toxic Plant)

Different varieties of yew are commonly cultivated including Taxus baccata, Taxus canadensis and Taxus cuspidata. It is commonly known as ground hemlock. All parts of the yew are toxic but poisoning with yew berries is uncommon. Toxane alkaloids are cardotonic and cardiotoxic. Irritant effect is due to presence of oils.

Symptoms

Vomiting, abdominal pain with diarrhoea, convulsions, impairment of consciousness, respiratory depression, complete heart block, broad complex bradycardia with profound hypotension. Ventricular tachycardia and fibrillation can cause sudden death.

Management

If more than two and three berries are ingested— gastric emptying has a role if performed within 4 hours of ingestion.

Cardiac pacing and inotropic support may be necessary if serious bradycardia develops.

Fab digoxin fragment antibodies can be tried.

Z

ZIDOVUDINE (Anti HIV)

It is used to treat AIDS and toxicity is possible due to overdose.

Symptoms

Ataxia, nystagmus, convulsions, minor increase in transaminase activity, leukopenia, thrombocytopenia with reduction in red cell counts.

Management

Activated charcoal: Repeated administration of 70-100 gm of slurry of activated charcoal to be given.

Diazepam is given to control convulsions.

Adult: 5-10 mg intravenous administration of undiluted diazepam over a period of 2-3 minutes.

Children: 0.25-0.4 mg/kg intravenous slowly over a period of 2-3 minutes is required.

Patency of airway should be adequately maintained and if necessary patient should be provided with ventilator.

APPENDIX

DRUGS OF ADDICTION WITH POPULAR NAMES

I. **Phencyclidine** is sold/available for use by addicts under different names such as **Aurora borealis, Angel dust Cycline, Crystal joints, Crystal, Chinese rhock, Embalming fluid, elephant or money tranquilliser. Mish peae Kill, peace weed, supergrass, super joint, super cool, surfer, Rocket fuel, sherman, snorts, scuffle, soma, TAC, TIC, white powder and zoom.**

II. **Cannabis** is called **Bhang, Bush, Dope, Durban poison, Ganja Grass, Hagga, Hash (Cannabis rein). Hash oil (Cannabis oil), Joint, Joy sticks, Marijuana, Mary Jane, MJ, Paki, Pot, Puff, Reefer, Resin (Cannabis resin), shirt, smoke, split, tea, Thai, sticks and weed.**

III. Addicts refer to **LDS** as **Acid, Beast, Blotter acid, Blue caps, Blue drops, Brown caps, Dome dots, Domes, Dots, Ghost, Green caps, Hawk, Microdots, Orange wedges, Paper acid, Pink drops, Purple haze, Purple wedges, Sunshine, White lightening, Windowpanes, Yellow caps and Yellow drops.**

IV. **Cocaine** by addicts is referred to as **bernice blow, C, cadillac of drugs, Charlie, Coke, dama blanca, dose, dynamite, flake, Gold dust, Green gold, Happy dust, Happy trails, Hocus, Ice, Jam, Lady, Leaf, Line, Pump's drug, Snort, snow, Speedball (Cocaine with heroin), Star spangled powder and Toot.**

V. **Amphetamine** by addicts is referred to as—**A, Adam (methylenedroxy amphetamine). Amphet, Bennees, Blues, Poorman's speed ball, Speed (amphetamine with other stimulants), speed for lovers, STP (dimethoxy methyl amphetamine), Sulph, Uppers, Wake ups, and Yuppie psychedelic (methylene dioxymethyl amphetamine).**

VI. **Heroin:** The most popular opioid in addict market is available under the following names: **Black tar, Boy, Brown Sugar, Chinese, Chinese rock, Elephant, H, Harry, Horse, Joy powder, Junk, Mexican Brown, Persian, Rock 'n' roll, Rufees, Smack, Stuff,**

Thing, TNT, White elephant, White junk and White snuff.

VII. **Methadone** the long acting synthetic opioid is sold in addict market under following names. **Dolli, Dolie Dolly, Dulophine.**

VIII. **Morphine:** The oldest addicting product by addicts is referred to as—**Cube juice, Dream, Hard stuff, Hocus, M, Muss, Emma, Monkey, Morf and Morpho.**

IX. **Fentanyl:** One of the most potent opioid is sold in addict markets as **China white X Barbiturates**—The hypnotics are no more popular with addicts yet a low percentage of addicts continue to abuse this group. Phenobarbitone is referred by addict as **Nembies and Downers.**

FEW POISONS WITH THEIR FATAL DOSES AND FATAL PERIODS

Poison	*Fatal dose*	*Fatal period*
Sulphuric acid	5-10 ml	12-24 hrs
Nitric acid	10-15 ml	12-24 hrs
Hydrochloric acid	15-20 ml	18-24 hrs
Oxalic acid	15-20 mgs	1-2 hrs
Phenol	1-2 gms	1-2 hrs
KOH/NaOH	5 gms	24 hrs
Sodium carbonate	30 gms	24 hrs
Potassium carbonate	18 gms	24 hrs
Ammonia	30 gms	24 hrs
Formaldehyde	30-90 ml	1-2 days
Iodine	2-4 gms	1-many days
Bromide	30-45 gms	6-18 hrs
Fluoride	5 mg/KBW	
Chloride	1000 ppm	5 min within 48 hrs
Phosphorus	60-120 mgs	2-8 days
Zn P	5 gms	24 hrs
Aluminium phosphide	0.15-0.5 gms	1-100 hrs
Sodium nitrate	1-2 gms	Few hrs
Glycerol nitrate	200 mgs	Few days
Barium chloride	1 gms	12 hrs
Arsenic	100-200 mgs	1-2 days
Mecury	1-4 gms	3-5 days

Contd...

Contd...

Poison	*Fatal dose*	*Fatal period*
Lead acetate	20 gms	1-2 days
Lead carbonate	4 (30) gms	1-2 days
Copper	15 gms	1-3 days
Copper sulphate	15-30 gms	1-3 days
Potassium permanganate	10-20 gms	Few hrs
Antimony: Tartar enetic	0.5-1 gms	24 hrs
Antimony trichloride	0.1-0.2 gms	24 hrs
Ricin communis	10 seeds	2-many days
	6 mgs	2-many days
Croton tigilum	4 seeds	6 hrs-3 days
	1.5 ml	6 hrs-3 days
Abrus injection	90-120 mgs	3-5 days
Oral	10 gms	3-5 days
Ergot	1-2 gms	1-many days
Calotrophis		
Semecarpus	5-10 gms	12-24 hrs
Catharides	15-50 mgs	24-36 hrs
Powder	1.5-3 gms	24-36 hrs
Opium	2 gms	6-12 hrs
Morphine	0.2 gms	6-12 hrs
Ethyl alcohol	150-200 ml	12-24 hrs
Methyl alcohol	60-240 ml	24-36 hrs
Lithium 3 to 4 nmol/L		
Barbiturates short acting	1-2 gms (3)	1-2 days
Medium acting	2-3 gms (7)	1-2 days
Long acting	3-5 gms (10)	1-2 days
Chloral hydrate	5-10 gms	8-12 hrs
Petroleum distillates hydrocarbons	15-50 ml	24 hrs
TEPP IM	50 mgs	½-4 hrs
Oral	100 mgs	½-4 hrs
OMPA/Parathion IM	80 mgs	½-4 hrs
Oral	175 mgs	½-4 hrs
HEPT IM	60 mgs	½-4 hrs
Oral	350 mgs	½-4 hrs
Malathion/Diazion oral	1 gm	½-4 hrs
Paraquat	3-5 gms	3-5 days
Organochlorines DDT	10 gms	
Gammexane	15 gms	
Endrin	5-6 gms	
Dinitro compounds	1-2 gms	4-15 days

Contd...

Contd...

Poison	*Fatal dose*	*Fatal period*
Datura	0.6-1 gms	24 hrs
	100-125 seeds	24 hrs
Cannabis charas	2/KBW mgs	Many days
Ganja	8/KBW mgs	Many days
Bhang	10/KBW mgs	Many days
Cocaine	1-1.5 gms	Few hrs
LSD	14 mgs	
Strychinne	15-50 mgs	1-2 hrs
Hydrocyanic acid	50-60 mgs	2-10 min
Sodium cyanide (1:500)	200-300 mgs	2-10 min
Aconite	1-2 mgs	1-8 hrs
Aconite root	1-2 gms	1-8 hrs
Croton oil	4-5 seeds	6 hrs-3 days
	1.5 ml	6 hrs-3 days
Calotrophis	Uncertain	12 hrs
Plumbagao zeylanica	Uncertain	Few days
Aspirin	5-10 gms	Few min to hrs
Salicylate	30 gms	
Antofebrin (Acetanilide)	15	Uncertain
Paracetamol	10-20 gms	2-4 days
Paraldehyde	100-150 Ml	12-24 hrs
Curare	30-60 mg	1-2 hrs
Tobacco	15-30 gms	5-15 min
Nicotin	60-100 mgs	5-15 min
Digitalis purpura	15-20 gms	1-24 hrs
Digoxin	4 mgs	
Nerium oduram (White)	15-20 gms	24-36 hrs
Cerebra thevetia (Yellow)	15-20 gms	½-1 hr
	8-10 seeds	½-1 hr
Cerebra odallum	1 kernel	1-2 days
Quinine	8-10 gms	2 hrs-2 days
Snakes	**Fatal mg**	
	Bite	
Cobra	12 200	
Russel	15 150	
Echis	8 5	
Krait	6 20	
CO_2	60-80%	
Mushroom	Uncertain	24 hrs

Fatal Doses

Chemical/Drug	*Lethal dose*	*Fatal period*
Sulfuric acid	10-15 ml	
Nitric acid	10-15 ml	
Hydrochloric acid	15-20 ml	
Mydrofluoric acid	Unclear	
Carbolic acid	10-15 gm or ml	
Oxalic acid	15-20 gm	
Salicylic acid	70-80 gm	
– Sodium salicylate and Acetyl salicylic acid	15-20 gm	
– Methyl salicylate	10-20 ml	
Ammonia	Gaseous-0.5% in air liquid-10-20 ml	
Sodium, Potassium and Ca Carbonate	Varies widely i.e. 5-20 gm	
Irritant Poisons		
Phosphorus	1 mg/kg (60-120 gm)	
Iodine	3-4 gm	
Metallic Irritants		
Arsenic Lead	200-250 mg	
Lead	20 gm of lead acetate	
Mercory (quick silver)	1-2 gm of meraric chloride	
Iron	200 m/kg of demental i rcu	
Copper	30 gm ($CuSO_4$)	
Thallium	1 gm	
Plant Origins		
Ricinos communis (castor or mole bean)	50-10 seeds/1 mg/kg (orally)	
Croton tiglium (croton)	5-6 seeds/1-2 ml of oil	
Abrus Precatorius	1-2 seeds/90-120 mg of abrin	
Bead or Indiaņ	(Jequirity or Rosary liquarice)	

Contd...

Contd...

Chemical/Drug	*Lethal dose*	*Fatal period*
Semecarpus anacardium (marking not)	10 gms	
Calotropis (madar)	Not known	
Capsicum (Chilli, cayenne pepper)	Not fatalities known	
Cerebral Poisons		
Opium (crude)	500 mg	
Morphine	200 mg	
Pethidine	1000 mg	
Codeine	800 mg (oral)	
Methadone	100 mg	
Heroin	50 mg	
Pentazocine	300 mg	
Propoxypnene	1000 mg (oral)	
Diphenoxylate	200 mg (oral)	
Ethyl alcohol	500-1000 ml of strong distilled spirit	
Isopropyl alcohol (Isopropanol)	200 mg%	
Ethylene glycol		
Methanol (Methyl alcohol wood alcohol)		
Barbiturates	1 gm, 2 gm and 3 gm of short acting, intermediate acting and long acting harbitortes respectively	
Chloral hydrate	7-10 gm	
Parathion	100 mg	
TEPP (Tetra ethyll pyro phosphate) (Octamethyl pyro phospharamide)	100 mg	
Malatnion	1 gm	
Diazinar	1 gm	
Organochlorines (Aldrin, chlordane, dieldrin, endosulfan)	2-6 gm	

Contd...